Navigating Breast Cancer: A Guide for the Newly Diagnosed

Lillie D. Shockney, RN, BS, MAS

*University Distinguished Service
Assistant Professor of Breast Cancer
Administrative Director
Johns Hopkins Avon Foundation
Breast Center*

JONES AND BARTLETT PUBLISHERS

Sudbury, Massachusetts

BOSTON   TORONTO   LONDON   SINGAPORE

World Headquarters

Jones and Bartlett Publishers
40 Tall Pine Drive
Sudbury, MA 01776
978-443-5000
info@jbpub.com
www.jbpub.com

Jones and Bartlett Publishers
Canada
6339 Ormindale Way
Mississauga, Ontario L5V 1J2
Canada

Jones and Bartlett Publishers
International
Barb House, Barb Mews
London W6 7PA
UK

Jones and Bartlett's books and products are available through most bookstores and online booksellers. To contact Jones and Bartlett Publishers directly, call 800-832-0034, fax 978-443-8000, or visit our website, www.jbpub.com.

Substantial discounts on bulk quantities of Jones and Bartlett's publications are available to corporations, professional associations, and other qualified organizations. For details and specific discount information, contact the special sales department at Jones and Bartlett via the above contact information or send an email to specialsales@jbpub.com.

Library of Congress Cataloging-in-Publication Data

Shockney, Lillie, 1953-
 Navigating breast cancer : a guide for the newly diagnosed / Lillie Shockney.
  p. cm.
 Includes bibliographical references and index.
 ISBN-13: 978-0-7637-4128-0 (alk. paper)
 ISBN-10: 0-7637-4128-0 (alk. paper)
 1. Breast--Cancer--Popular works. I. Title.
 RC280.B8S4952 2007
 616.99'449--dc22
                                    2006016492
6048

Production Credits

Executive Publisher, Medicine: Chris Davis
Production Director: Amy Rose
Associate Editor: Kathy Richardson
Production Editor: Carolyn F. Rogers
Associate Marketing Manager: Laura Kavigian
Manufacturing Buyer: Therese Connell
Composition: Northeast Compositors, Inc.
Cover Design: Timothy Dziewit
Cover Art: © Image Club Graphics
Section Opener Art: © Image Club Graphics
Printing and Binding: Malloy, Inc.
Cover Printing: Malloy, Inc.

Printed in the United States of America
12 11 10 09 08   10 9 8 7 6 5

Contents

So you've recently been diagnosed with breast cancer. . . .

Know that you are not alone and do not have to make this journey alone through treatment—there are more than 2 million women in the United States today who can confidently say they are breast cancer survivors. I am among those 2 million.

A woman's greatest fear is hearing the news, "You have breast cancer." For decades this has been true. And though more women will be diagnosed with cardiovascular disease, that disorder doesn't shake women's foundation like breast cancer. Our brain goes numb, and, in a split second, we feel as if our life is completely out of control. I know. I'm a nurse who cares for women with this disease, and I'm a breast cancer survivor myself, having been diagnosed at the age of 38 in 1992. I am now healthier than I've ever been in my life, and life is good.

Although you, as the woman, are the one diagnosed with the disease, everyone who loves you is affected by it. Your loved ones can play a critical role in your transformational journey from breast cancer victim to breast cancer survivor.

From knowledge comes power. This book is designed to empower you with information so you can participate confidently in the planning of your treatment. Gaining an understanding about the treatment of breast cancer and the choices you have in planning that treatment will help reduce your anxiety and help you regain a sense of control.

No matter what your specific circumstances, I hope this book will help you embark on what will become known as a life-altering experience. Consider me part of your support team as you begin and continue on this journey, until it is behind you. Think of me as part of your cheering squad (and yes, I do have pink pom-poms).

—Lillie Shockney

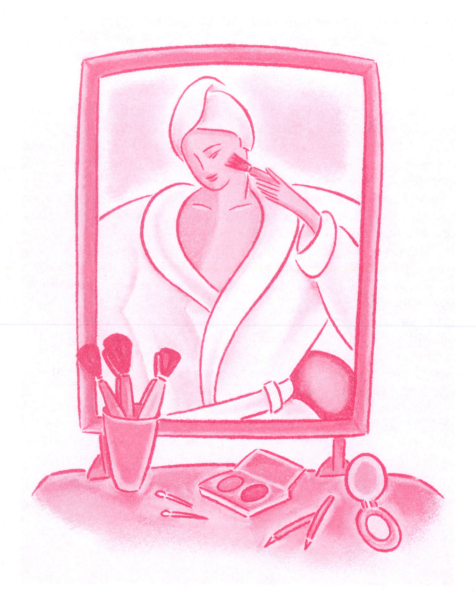

Let's Get Started

Chapter 1

The Decision-Making Process

"All I can think about is 'I have breast cancer.'"

I felt overwhelmed when I was diagnosed. I wasn't sure if I wanted to rewind the videotape of my life and slow it down or fast-forward it to quickly see if I made out okay or not.

I had a wonderful mentor to reflect on, Miss Bertha, a family friend, who learned she had advanced breast cancer four decades ago, when medicine had little to offer women for treatment. Despite being given a terrible prognosis (she was told she would live less than 5 months) she beat the odds. She taught me the value of combining good medical treatment with being optimistic, getting lots of support, laughing every day to build her immune system, and developing new personal goals for herself. Her first new goal, she said, was to outlive her doctor—and she did! She lived for 21 more years!

As an oncology nurse for 30 years and Administrative Director of the Johns Hopkins Avon Foundation Breast Center, I devote all of my time professionally and personally to helping newly diagnosed women navigate through their breast cancer treatment. No two patients are alike. Each has different levels of understanding, methods to use to participate in the decision making, and attitudes as to how they want to approach this experience. As a patient advocate and health care professional, I want the best outcome for each woman. As a survivor, I want her beside me in years to come celebrating her survivorship at a breast cancer event like the Avon 2-Day Walk.

—*Lillie Shockney*

Preconceived Ideas About Breast Cancer

Breast cancer is the disease most feared by women. Often, women fear losing their breasts, their hair, and of course, their lives. For many, this disease has a strong association with a loss of femininity and womanhood.

Previous experience with others who have had the disease, both survivors and those who didn't survive, greatly influences how people think about breast cancer and their own ability to overcome it. Keep in mind that science is moving at a rapid pace and that, blessedly, new discoveries are happening very rapidly in the field of breast cancer diagnosis and treatment. So, if you know someone who was treated more than a decade ago, understand that the treatment plan may be very different today—and less traumatic for you.

An effective way to regain control of your life—and your health—is to empower yourself with information about breast cancer and its treatment. Information is power, and with it you will be better prepared to embark on the decision-making process that lies before you. A great deal of information is available to help educate you and your loved ones about the disease and the latest treatments available.

Before embarking on any treatment, talk extensively with your medical team and ask a lot of questions. Although medical advice from family members and friends is meant to be helpful, it may add to the stress you are experiencing. Rely on the health care team of professionals (doctors, nurses, social workers, counselors). They are experienced and can guide women to the medical information and treatment options that will work best for your specific breast cancer diagnosis. Let's first review a few facts about breast cancer to put you in a positive frame of mind and to get you started with the learning process.

Your chances of survival are excellent. Based on statistics, more than 85 percent of the women diagnosed with breast cancer this year will join the group of more than 2 million survivors of the disease who are alive and active today in the United States. For women who are diagnosed and treated early, if the cancer is confined to the breast ducts alone, we can even use the word "cured."

In most cases, you won't have to make snap decisions about treatment. Women can take several weeks to choose doctors and decide on the appropriate course of action. Though you just learned that the cancer is there, in most cases, it has been there for several years to become a 1 centimeter mass on a mammogram. Time is still on your side to make educated decisions that are in your best interest. Fast is not better in this situation.

Here are some more facts about breast cancer:

- Greater than 80 percent of women are good candidates for breast-conserving surgery (lumpectomy) and don't have to lose their breasts to this disease (*Johns Hopkins University*).

- Research shows that women who seek emotional support during and after treatment have higher survival rates than those who decline to do so (*Stanford School of Medicine*).

- Generally, the earlier you are diagnosed, the less treatment you will need to become a long-term survivor.

- The side effects from adjuvant treatment (chemotherapy and radiation) can be minimized with the use of drugs now available for that purpose.

• Many women report that their lives are more fulfilling after a diagnosis of breast cancer than they were before.

• Seventy percent of women diagnosed with breast cancer have no known risk factors for getting the disease.

• Approximately 12 percent of women diagnosed with breast cancer have a family history of the disease.

• The majority of women work and continue their activities of daily living during treatment.

It is extremely important that you feel confident in the health care team taking care of you. Surgeons who specialize in breast cancer surgery provide you the recommendations as to what type of breast cancer surgery is best for your situation and perform the surgical procedure (refer to Chapter 5); medical oncologists evaluate your case and provide recommendations as well as oversee the administration of chemotherapy, targeted therapy (refer to Chapter 8), and hormonal therapy (refer to Chapter 6); radiation oncologists evaluate your treatment needs related to radiation and administer radiation therapy (refer to Chapter 6). Not all patients need all the various types of treatment. Some may only have surgery. Others may have surgery and radiation only. Still others may have the above along with chemotherapy, targeted therapy and hormonal therapy. When chemotherapy, targeted therapy, radiation therapy and hormonal therapy are used for women who do not appear to have had the breast cancer spread elsewhere in their body, this type of treatment is referred to as adjuvant therapy. It's being given as a way to prevent recurrence of the disease and not for the purpose of actually treating breast cancer that has spread. The most common sequence for treatment is surgery, followed by chemotherapy, then radiation, then targeted therapy and hormonal therapy, if needed. There is a paradigm shift happening, however, to do chemotherapy first, then surgery, and other adjuvant therapy afterwards. This type of treatment is referred to as neoadjuvant chemotherapy. It depends on your specific situation as to what will be recommended.

Recent studies at Northwestern University have confirmed that women who go to a facility that performs a relatively high volume of breast treatments on the average have better clinical outcomes and higher survival rates. So, if at all possible, seek out a facility and health care team that specializes in breast cancer treatment. (See Chapter 2, "Features of a Breast Center.")

After selecting the facility and the doctors for your treatment, make a list of questions to ask when you go for appointments. It is advisable that you take someone you trust with you. Two sets of eyes and ears are better than one. Take a tape recorder, too. That little machine can be a blessing because when you are under stress, it is hard to recall information and things easily can be misinterpreted.

Physicians usually prefer that the patient be the individual asking the questions because that is the person who will be undergoing treatment. Your loved one is there for support and to ask additional questions that may be prompted as part of the discussion. As the patient, you should feel that you are part of the health care team. Treatment is to be planned with you—not for you. Remember, patient empowerment is important.

Also, educate your doctors and nurses about who you are. You are not just a woman with breast cancer; you are a mother, career woman, Girl Scout leader, Sunday school teacher, wife, mountain climber, type A personality, worrywart. Your doctors need to see you as a total picture in order to help plan the best treatment with you. You are more than a patient. You are a person with a life that is on hold right now.

Ask for copies of your medical records. Specific items to request include the pathology report, the mammography report, any other X-rays such as ultrasound or CAT scans, and operative reports.

Chapter 2

Features of a Breast Center

"You have time to make sure you are in good hands."

One of the challenges for consumers today is knowing whether they are being cared for in a breast center or merely a facility that calls itself a breast center. Unfortunately, there are no standards that define what is meant by this term. Those of us working in this field for decades believe we know what the features, services, and components should be, but our definition is not universally applied. Ideally, a breast center would be part of a comprehensive cancer center designated by the National Cancer Institute (NCI); however, not all breast centers are. Seeking a facility and team that has the programs, services, features and clinical expertise you need is important and should be your focus in deciding where to go for your care. The following sections list some of the features to look for. You are seeking a total program of care, not piecemeal treatment.

Easy Access

If you have been advised that you have breast cancer you will want an appointment as soon as possible—not because it is an emergency, but because until you have a plan of action you will feel out of control and in a state of limbo, a very uncomfortable place to be.

Until you are seen by a breast surgeon and have answers about your clinical situation, your anxiety and stress level will remain high. Most breast centers, in acknowledgment of this, will (and should) schedule you for an appointment within 48 hours of your call or doctor's referral. Fear of the unknown is the worst fear of all. Even if the news you receive is bad, you can take comfort in knowing that now you can begin working with the doctors to plan what will be the best treatment choices for you.

Patient Empowerment

It is important that you be given the knowledge you need to enable you to actively participate in decisions about your care and treatment. Some physicians are reluctant to empower women in this way. It is a patient's right, and should be a key factor in deciding where you want to receive your treatment.

Patient (and Family) Education

Not only do you need to be educated about breast cancer, the treatment options, and what to expect each step along the way, but so do important members of your family. This requires an investment of time and resources by the health care professionals taking care of you. You want to receive and be educated about your treatment plans as thoroughly as possible. You need to have easy access to someone in the breast center who you can feel comfortable asking questions of and feel confident in their responses. By doing so you will come to understand what is happening to your body and what needs to be done to get you well again. Your family members who love you and need to support you benefit from this education too, because they worry about you. They need to understand what is happening so they can devote their time and energy to emotionally supporting you.

Multidisciplinary Case Conferences

A key advantage to having a multidisciplinary team approach is the special expertise each health care professional offers to each patient's unique situation. Centers that hold weekly breast cancer case conferences (sometimes referred to as "tumor boards") to discuss in detail a patient's clinical condition, diagnostic findings, and recommendations for optimal treatment are beneficial to the patient's overall well-being and clinical outcome. This is a way to help ensure that the patient is being given individualized attention and care by utilizing maximum breast cancer knowledge, experience, and expertise by the breast center team. Such case conferences are attended by breast surgeons, medical oncologists, radiation oncologists, pathologists, genetics experts, plastic surgeons, oncology nurses and sometimes even social workers. Cases that are more complex are commonly presented by the physician who saw the patient in consultation and the doctor at this time requests the team to provide input regarding the treatment plan that would be best to recommend for the patient. The pathology slides are viewed by the team on a large screen while the pathologist describes the pathology results. The radiologist displays the mammograms, ultrasound, and any other scans or breast imaging studies that have been performed and discusses the findings seen on each of them. Then the doctors discuss the case openly to determine what would be the best treatment strategy to recommend. The physician who presented the case is responsible to contact the patient afterward and let her know what the results were of this discussion.

Special Breast Imaging Services
Appointments Right Away

If a woman is being referred by her family doctor or gynecologist for evaluation of a suspicious lump or other potentially serious breast abnormality (like an inverted nipple that is new) she wants to know right away if it is cancer. For that matter, if she finds the lump herself she doesn't want there to be any delay in getting answers about her situation. Mammography facilities should offer appointments for such patients as quickly as possible. Ideally, the patient would be seen within a few days of the referral being made.

Often radiologists are not readily available to read the films and talk with the patient about what the mammogram showed. Ideally you want to go to a facility that has radiologists who specialize in breast imaging and are available to read the films while you are there and most importantly tell you what they show. Be sure to call and ask whether they offer this type of clinical service. It is one additional way to reduce your anxiety and speed the process along for you to get answers and proceed with treatment if it is determined to be cancer. If they do not have a dedicated radiologist for reading breast imaging studies like mammograms and ultrasounds, ask what steps are taken to ensure accuracy such as a second reading of the films by another radiologist who serves as a quality control step. Some breast imaging facilities use electronic technology for doing this type of "second reading" which has proven helpful too. A computer is trained to look for abnormalities on the mammogram and flags tiny areas that warrant further evaluation by the radiologist.

Mammography and Diagnostic Evaluation in Breast Imaging Setting

Mammography remains the gold standard for screening for early stage breast cancer. There are mammography facilities that are located within and are part of a Breast Center and there are mammography facilities that are free standing facilities and operate independently. Most perform both screening mammograms for women having annual mammograms and are symptom free of a breast abnormality, as well as offer diagnostic mammograms for women who have some type of breast symptom that warrants further investigation and evaluation to determine what it is. Most also provide breast ultrasound that enables the breast tissue to be viewed using sonography rather than X-ray and can be helpful in distinguishing between a solid mass (benign or malignant tumors) and a liquid mass (cysts). Most facilities are still using traditional analog film mammography which means that the breast X-ray is captured on X-ray film.

There is a movement happening now to have more facilities switch over to a computerized way of capturing mammography images. Studies have confirmed that women who are premenopausal and have dense breast tissue on analog film mammography can benefit by having their mammogram captured digitally as a computer image. A tumor is white on a mammogram and for women with dense breast tissue density also appears white. This can result in the radiologist trying to distinguish between subtle differences in whiteness which sometimes is simply not possible. Capturing the breast imaging digitally enables the radiologist to lighten and darken the background on the monitor and sometimes find masses that otherwise may go unnoticed until a later time. Ask if you meet these criteria for needing more detailed imaging and whether digital mammography is available at that facility.

Percutaneous Biopsy—Minimally Invasive Stereotactic Breast Biopsy, Core Biopsy, and Fine Needle Biopsies

Four types of biopsy procedures can now be done in breast imaging/mammography if the facility has the technology and medical expertise. A stereotactic biopsy involves having the patient lay on a table on her abdomen with her breast that is to be biopsied dropped through a hole in the table. The breast is compressed in mammography paddles and a mammogram image is projected on a computer screen. The computer provides information about the exact location of the abnormality to be biopsied. A large gauge needle connected to a special machine designed to take samples of the breast tissue is used for obtaining the biopsy specimen. Usually several samples are taken and are X-rayed to ensure that the tissue targeted for evaluation was adequately sampled. This is commonly done when the abnormality is microcalcifications or a tiny mass that cannot be felt by the doctor and only can be seen on mammography. Core biopsies are done usually in breast ultrasound when the breast abnormality can best be seen and felt in ultrasound. This involves taking a large gauge needle and inserting it into the center of the mass and tissue is removed for pathology to evaluate. The third minimally invasive technique is called a fine needle biopsy. This is done for masses that can be easily felt by the doctor. He or she inserts a smaller gauge needle and only removes a few cells from the mass for the pathologist to review under the microscope. In each of these three methods, local anesthesia is commonly used to numb the area. These methods of doing breast biopsies enable the patient to have a sample of tissue removed without having an open biopsy requiring an incision. Having the biopsy done as a stereotactic or core biopsy requires special equipment and devices that not all mammography facilities currently have. It also requires special credentialling for the radiologist doing this type of procedure. Learning about these programs and services is an additional way to judge how up to date the facility is that you are considering going to for your care. Today more than 90 percent of biopsies can be performed in this manner with results back from pathology the next day. The fourth way of biopsy is an open excisional biopsy. This is performed by a breast surgeon and is done in the operating room. This may be necessary if the abnormality is close to the chest wall or for some other reason a radiologist has recommended that it be peformed in this manner rather than as a stereotactic, core, or fine needle biopsy in breast imaging.

Inform the Patient and Referring Physician of the Findings Right Away

Once you have had a biopsy, you want to know the results as soon as possible. Check to see what the turn-around time is for pathology results. Many facilities can tell you or your doctor the results of a biopsy within 24 hours. The sooner you know what you are dealing with the sooner you can begin to make plans about the best treatment options for you to pursue.

Clinical Trials

Having the opportunity to have available to you as many treatment options as possible is important. Hospitals who participate in clinical trials usually can offer more innovative treatment options. In some cases the treatments being studied in these clinical trials are very new and the medical field is still learning about all of their full benefits, value, and risks. It can include drugs that are not FDA approved yet with the goal that the results of the clinical trials will determine the potential benefits that could lead to FDA approval. If you are asked to participate in such a trial you are paving the way for the development of innovative research that could make an important impact on other women diagnosed in the future with breast cancer. You are also being closely monitored throughout your treatment process so that data can be collected about your experience with the chemotherapy agents you've been given. You might also be asked to participate in a study that already has proven to be beneficial for treating breast cancer for some patients, and now different dosages are being tested to determine the optimal dosage and frequency for you and other patients treated in the future. These new discoveries not only benefit you today, but also will make a big difference in how many lives we save from breast cancer in the future. Not all clinical trials will be of benefit to the specific patient participating in them since every patient is different. It is advantageous to participate, however, looking at the big picture for the development of innovative treatments of the future that may replace current treatments or complement them.

Full Range of Surgical Options

It is very important to have breast cancer surgery done by a surgeon who performs a large volume of breast cancer surgery. (Note I said breast *cancer* surgeries, not breast surgeries.) It is preferable that the surgeon be someone who specializes in breast cancer. Studies have been published confirming that survival rates are higher for patients receiving surgical management by breast surgeons who do perform high volumes of breast cancer surgery. The doctors who you are considering to take care of you should have clinical quality outcomes data that describe their patients' length of time in the hospital on average for women having breast cancer surgery with and without reconstruction, complications that occur during or after surgery, and satisfaction data from prior patients' experiences. All of this is important information when choosing who you want to have take care of you.

Ask what type of preoperative teaching is offered for patients and their families as well. Usually a breast center might have dedicated nurses to provide education to patients so that they are well prepared for the type of surgery they are to have, thereby reducing anxiety prior to and at the time of surgery.

You also have the right to state-of-the-art surgical options. More than 80 percent of women are good candidates for breast conservation surgery today (lumpectomy). Sentinel node biopsy is also a standard of care now, enabling the surgeon to identify the guard node and remove only that single node to assess if the cancer has spread. This dramatically reduces the risk of lymphedema, a major concern of women having axillary node dissections. Women needing mastectomy or desiring this as their surgical option also have the right to a full spectrum of reconstruction options. Not all options are available at all breast centers, however. You may need to travel elsewhere to receive surgeries, such as deep inferior epigastric perforator (DIEP) artery flap or superior gluteal artery perforator (S-GAP) that require use of a microscope for reconnecting blood vessels, spare all your muscles, and result in a transplantation of fat from your tummy or buttocks to rebuild your breast. This combined with skin-sparing mastectomy offers women cosmetic results far superior to what was available in past years. It also reduces the risk of hernia, bulge, and other complications more commonly found with trans-rectus abdominis muscle (TRAM) flap surgeries. This portion of your surgery would be performed by a plastic surgeon who specializes in breast reconstruction. Again, you want someone who has done a large volume of the type of reconstruction you are interested in receiving. Also ask to review this surgeon's clinical outcomes data for results and look at photographs of before and after pictures of other patients.

Medical Oncology

Most, but not all, patients diagnosed with breast cancer need some form of chemotherapy as part of their treatment. Again, most breast centers offer such clinical care. Make sure that the medical oncologist who is overseeing your treatment specializes in the treatment of breast cancer—someone who treats a large volume of women with this disease and has access to a spectrum of clinical trials. You want to have a medical oncologist who is readily accessible in the event you need to talk with him or her urgently while going through treatment. Ask questions about the doctor's procedure for addressing emergency calls as well as what type of monitoring will be done while you are undergoing adjuvant therapy (additional treatment given to prevent recurrence of the disease). Ask about the survival statistics for breast cancer patients treated at the facility you are considering, too. All cancer patients' data are entered into a national database, giving cancer specialists the ability to compare various treatment modalities and clinical outcomes. Hospitals who treat large volumes of cancer patients also study their own data and compare them to national statistics. You want to be in the hands of a team of professionals who have a history of good outcomes.

Ask what education is available to help you prepare for known side effects of treatment, and for information about getting fitted for a wig as well as skin care needs that may occur during treatment. Some breast centers offer these services within their facility.

Hormonal therapy is also something that a medical oncologist may discuss with a patient. A special pathology test is done to determine if the cancer cells are stimulated to grow from exposure to estrogen. When they are, hormonal therapy in the form of selective estrogen receptor modulators (SERMs) or aromatase inhibitors (AIs) may be recommended or discussed. If the pathology results confirm that the cancer cells are "hormone receptor positive" then it is likely that a discussion about hormonal therapy will take place. This therapy may last anywhere from 2 to 10 years, so how you will be followed and monitored for side effects during this long period is important to discuss. For women coping with metastatic disease or the return of the breast cancer, they may be given a special type of hormonal therapy that works by blocking estrogen's binding ability; this is called an estrogen down regulator.

Targeted biologic therapy is now available. For women who have a specific prognostic factor called HER2neu which is confirmed to be positive (referred to as being "+++," or "three plus"), the medical oncologist may recommend targeted biological therapy in the form of Herceptin (trastuzumab). This therapy is administered intravenously on a specific schedule several times a month for approximately a year and has proven or been shown to reduce risk of the breast cancer recurring in the future when combined with standard adjuvant chemotherapy and radiation or hormonal therapy when appropriate. It is considered to also be adjuvant therapy. There are also situations in which targeted biologic therapy is used to treat advanced or metastatic HER2neu positive breast cancers as well.

Radiation Oncology

Patients who undergo lumpectomy for treatment of their breast cancer almost always receive radiation afterwards. Many hospitals offer radiation oncology services. If the type of treatment that is advised for you includes radiation therapy, you will want to ask questions about the radiation oncology physician's experience with treating breast cancer patients. Again, it is valuable to go to a facility that has extensive experience with treating this specific type of cancer. As is the case with all your treatment, you as a patient should be given the opportunity to participate in the decision making about this type of treatment option.

There are different methods of delivering radiation for breast cancer treatment today. Some are part of clinical trials and other techniques are the current standard of care. Ask about your options and statistics related to local recurrence rates for each.

Also inquire about how your heart and lungs will be protected from the radiation field. Today a device called an Active Breath Control Device is available at some centers that provides an easy way for the patient's heart and lungs to be spared radiation by controlling her breathing during the actual radiation treatment.

Genetic Counseling

Genetic counseling is a special program for women who have a family history of breast cancer or have other factors that make them at higher risk for developing this disease. Counseling and genetic testing require specialists who not only are experts in this field, but also have excellent communication skills. The choice to have counseling and especially to decide to proceed with genetic testing is one to be taken seriously and with some caution. Though it may sound simple to be tested, there are many issues to consider before making such a choice. Physicians and nurses who have chosen to specialize in this field have expertise with helping women make these choices. If this is an area of interest to you or your family, you want to go to a facility that has many years of experience with genetic counseling and testing for breast cancer. Ask how long their program has existed and how many patients have been counseled and tested during that time. This will give you some idea as to their experience with this specialized type of service.

High-Risk Assessment for Breast Cancer

Being evaluated for your or a family member's risk of developing breast cancer may be important for you. There are health care professionals who specialize in this type of screening and evaluation. Ask the breast center where you are contemplating going for your care if they offer this service, who performs the service, and how many patients they screen a year. The program should be conducted by a doctor or a nurse practitioner who specializes in breast health screening programs.

Pathology Services

Patients don't always think about pathology, but it is a very important service. The pathologist who looks at your tissue specimen determines what type of breast cancer you have, how quickly it is growing, and whether it has spread to your lymph nodes, and provides other important pieces of clinical information to your breast surgeon, medical oncologist, and radiation oncologist. Accuracy and completeness are critical. Some say that the pathologist "holds all the cards" because his or her opinion about what is on your pathology slides determines your diagnosis and your treatment.

It is difficult for a layperson to assess whether the pathology services being provided at a hospital are of good quality. One source for this information is the Joint Commission for Accreditating Healthcare Organizations (JCAHO). It inspects hospitals on a tri-annual basis and records reports based on its findings. Included in its report are its findings for the pathology department. Although the inspectors don't actually look at slides and determine whether they were accurately interpreted, they do look at the processes used by pathology to determine how effectively they work. They also review the credential files of the pathologists and other faculty at the facility. You may wish to consider obtaining a second opinion about the pathology results by taking your pathology slides to a second facility that also has extensive experience in diagnosing and treating breast cancer.

The pathologist should be considered one of the members of the breast center team and actively participate in the case conferences referenced earlier in this document. The information he or she provides serves as the road map for determining the treatment plan options that are best for your specific situation. Ask if the pathologist attends these conferences and what role he or she plays in the actual case discussion. Ideally, the breast center will have a dedicated pathologist for review of breast tissue.

Continuity of Care

As more and more health care services are converted from an inpatient setting to an outpatient setting, the need to ensure effective and efficient continuity of care heightens. Ask the breast center faculty how they go about keeping your primary care doctor or referring physician aware of your condition and treatment status. Check to see how they keep track of how you are doing after you go home following surgery or chemotherapy treatments. Ask who is responsible for coordinating your care. You need to have confidence that you are being watched over even when you are not physically at the hospital. Some facilities have nurse practitioners who stay in touch with their patients via telephone once they are home. Some offer home health nursing care after surgical treatment is done. More are beginning to offer patient navigators to help with coordination of care. The team of professionals taking care of you also needs to stay in close contact with one another—that's why they are a team. Ask them how they communicate with one another and keep each other informed about your progress and needs. You want to be cared for by a team who stays well connected with you and with one another, including your referring physician or doctor who functions as your family doctor. Feeling confident that you are receiving good continuity of care provides wonderful peace of mind to you and your family.

Urgent Care Services

When an urgent problem arises, such as sickness that won't subside following a treatment, you need to have ready access to a professional who can take care of this situation promptly. Ask what the breast center's procedures are for handling such emergencies. A breast center needs to have a professional health care provider available for its patients 24 hours a day, 7 days a week to handle emergencies. In addition, the patients should be well informed about how to access this urgent care service and know they can confidently rely on it. If the center's patient education program has been thorough, you and your family will know how to take care of most crises and head them off at the pass (for example, taking an anti-nausea drug at a designated time to prevent vomiting later on). Unforeseen circumstances do arise on occasion, however, which warrant prompt intervention by a doctor or nurse. Knowing and understanding how urgent care needs such as these are handled is important. Though you may never need to use it, you want to know that such a program is in place and works well.

Continuing Education Programs and Seminars

When your treatment is over you will still want to stay "abreast" of the latest treatment programs and research discoveries being made about breast cancer. Your continued good health may depend on it. Most women thirst for information and want to learn as much as they can—it may make a difference for their own health or for someone in their family who they care about. Check to see what type of continuing educational programs the facility offers related to breast cancer. Examples of seminars that might be offered include new options for hormonal therapy, coping with menopausal symptoms, breast cancer gene research findings, the latest in breast reconstruction, and coping with fear of reoccurrence of breast cancer. Although your treatment may be over, the disease and its long-term effects may continue. You will want to stay informed and should expect the center where you received your care to help in keeping you updated at routine intervals.

Emotional Support

Though you will be relying on family and friends during this time, there are others who can greatly benefit you, too. These people are women who have experienced what you are about to embark upon. They are breast cancer survivor volunteers. Ask if the breast center offers a matching program so that you can talk with a survivor volunteer who had the same stage of disease and treatment plan as yourself. Though each of us are individuals and may have different personal experiences with the diagnosis and treatment process, talking with someone whose experience was similar to your situation can be comforting.

Chapter 3

Getting Started: Time for Your Initial Consultation

"I hope I remember all of my questions."

Usually the doctor who performed the biopsy will recommend a breast surgeon for you to see. You still have the right to obtain information about his or her credentials as well as the breast center he or she is recommending. It is not unusual for women to seek a second opinion after seeing the doctor as well. Most breast centers will require that you bring your pathology slides from the biopsy with you (or arrange for them to be shipped in advance) for their pathologist to review and verify the diagnosis. The doctor will also want to see your mammograms and any other breast imaging studies that have been performed.

You should expect your doctors and nurses to:

- Willingly answer your questions

- Help you understand information that is complicated for you

- Spend adequate time with you to address your questions and needs

- Respect your privacy and confidentiality

- Be sensitive

- Be skillful and knowledgeable

- Not discourage a second opinion

- Be supportive

- Engage you in a manner that helps you feel you are a member of your own health care team

Questions that many women want to ask the doctor at time of initial consultation include:

- Am I a candidate for breast-conserving surgery (lumpectomy)?

- What is my risk of recurrence if I have lumpectomy surgery vs. mastectomy?

- If I need chemotherapy, will I feel sick; if so, for how long?

- Are there breast cancer survivors here I can talk with who have had the same treatment I'm about to undergo? Do you offer a support group here for patients? How about for partners?

- Who do I call if I have questions after I leave today?

- What stage is my breast cancer, based on the information you have thus far?

- Can you translate the pathology report from my biopsy into layman's terms for me?

Some questions that women often have to consider are quite sensitive and require time and candor to discuss. For example, you may have been anticipating starting a family soon or adding to the family you currently have. Although there isn't a lot of information on the subject of pregnancy and breast cancer recurrence, your doctor may be able to give you some advice on this subject—but only if you tell him or her more about yourself and your desire to have children. Some treatments also may impact the ability to conceive in the future.

Another sensitive issue is the fact that your children, siblings, and mother all are now at a somewhat higher risk of developing breast cancer as a result of your own diagnosis. What can be done to help reduce their risk? How can you cope with the worry of potentially seeing a loved one also one day diagnosed with breast cancer? Will your doctor recommend genetic testing?

These are examples of issues to talk about and share with your health care team as well as to discuss as a family. The good news is that there are better methods being developed today for earlier and more accurate detection than ever before, and there are drug therapies and other treatments designed to reduce the risk of breast cancer occurring in women who are at high risk.

Often women try to figure out what caused their breast cancer. This will remain, for most, an unanswered question. The bottom line is that it usually isn't helpful to be doing an inventory of your life trying to decipher this question. It is smarter to move forward. Most risk factors are out of our control anyway, including beginning menstruation prior to age 12, having your first child after age 30, experiencing menopause after age 50, and having first-degree family relatives diagnosed with breast cancer. Potential factors that may contribute to risk and *are* within your control are smoking, alcohol consumption, taking hormone replacement therapy, weight gain, and lack of exercise.

Understanding Your Biopsy Report

Initially, all information printed on medical reports and told to you will sound Greek. By the end of your treatment you will be quoting this information yourself with confidence and knowledge. Some women say they think they can write their own encyclopedia on this disease when they finish. It's probably true. To jump start your knowledge base, let's begin with your pathology report from your biopsy. The majority of biopsies are done as core biopsies and provide a tiny window into the big picture to be uncovered soon. This piece of tissue provides information about the type of breast cancer you have and a few specifics about its characteristics. It isn't intended to tell much more than this. The surgery that will be performed will answer the other prognostic questions that need to be answered, so it can be premature to ask the doctor too much about your prognosis, the stage of the disease, and precisely what the details of your treatment will be. Putting together information from your breast imaging studies (mammograms, ultrasounds, and breast MRI if one happened to be done) along with the biopsy information provides what is needed to determine your surgical requirements.

There are two primary types of invasive breast cancer. You can research others that are diagnosed less frequently on Web sites like www.breastcancer.org or www.hopkinsbreastcenter.org, but for our purposes for now, let's stick with the major players: *invasive/ infiltrating ductal carcinoma* and *invasive/infiltrating lobular carcinoma*. Eighty-five percent of invasive cancers in the breast are ductal. This means that the disease started in the ducts of the breast and spread into the nearby fatty tissue of the breast. Invasive does not always mean it has spread elsewhere. Checking the lymph nodes and reviewing other prognostic factors during surgery help to determine the risk of this having happened. Invasive lobular carcinoma starts in the lobules of the breast and accounts for 12 percent of invasive breast cancers. The treatment for these is the same, no matter where they "started." Determining their actual size is done by pathology. The size of ductal carcinomas usually is fairly easy to estimate on mammograms or ultrasound. Lobular carcinomas, however, can be a little trickier and can be smaller or larger than what appears on an X-ray image. There are situations in which the pathology report will label the cells "mammary carcinoma." In this case, there is a mixture of ductal and lobular cancer cells.

There is also a type of breast cancer called noninvasive carcinoma. This is breast cancer at the earliest stage at which it can be found. It is known as *ductal carcinoma in situ* (DCIS). The ductal cancer cells are limited to the lining of the duct, remaining at their original site, and have not yet become invasive. This type of cancer usually cannot be felt as a lump and can be seen only on a mammogram. (It is a primary reason why women are encouraged to get annual mammograms—to find it at this stage.)

A point of confusion is with the term *lobular carcinoma in situ* (LCIS). Though the word *carcinoma* is used, it doesn't actually refer to cancer at all, but to a marker for predicting risk of developing breast cancer in the future. Women with this type of cell found on biopsy are usually referred to a high risk specialist for further evaluation and should not be told they have cancer, because it isn't cancer at all.

A rarer form of breast cancer is *inflammatory breast cancer*. The cancer cells are actually in the skin of the breast to start. The pathology report will usually say that there are "dermal lymphatic cells" in the cancer cells. This is known to be a more aggressive form of breast cancer and presents quite differently on clinical examination, usually with the presence of a rash on the breast and a normal mammogram.

The *grade of the cells* may also be recorded as part of the report. Grades are 1, 2, or 3.

- 1 = slow growing, and might be also referred to as "well differentiated" cells.

- 2 = average growing, and may be called "moderately differentiated cells."

- 3 = rapidly growing, and may be termed "poorly differentiated cells."

Don't be surprised if your report says grade 3. Some are. This doesn't mean to get a stethoscope and see if you can hear your breast cancer growing (as one patient told me she was doing). "Rapidly growing" is a relative term. In most cases, cancer has been there for some time. You are now aware it is there so it is an anxious time for you, but it has been working on getting itself established for probably several years. That's why it's important now to gather your information to make good decisions and not rush into anything without a solid knowledge base.

There are additional tests that are done on the breast cancer cells which are more commonly done on the breast cancer specimen removed at time of the lumpectomy or mastectomy surgery. Doing these prognostic tests on the "whole tumor" rather than on a tiny piece is usually preferred by the pathologist. These two prognostic tests are listed below.

The pathologist will also assess the cells to determine if they are stimulated to grow by estrogen or progesterone. This will be listed as hormone receptors or "ER/PR." Hormone receptor positive means that the cells were stimulated to grow by hormones. This is considered a favorable prognostic factor to have. Often this test won't be done until final pathology from the surgery specimen to help ensure its accuracy. Remember, the biopsy is a piece of the whole. So to ensure an adequate representation for prognostic factors used to determine your treatment, the pathologist may decide to sample a larger piece in pathology to determine this answer. For women who have hormone receptor positive breast cancers, it is relatively common for the oncologist to recommend hormonal therapy as part of the treatment.

An additional test to measure a prognostic factor called HER2neu receptor will also be performed by the pathologist if the cancer cells were invasive carcinoma. This is known as an oncogene measurement. The role of oncogenes is to control cell growth. Extra protein makes cells grow out of control. If the HER2 test is "positive" then it means that the cancer cells have too much HER2 receptor protein on the surface of the cell or there are extra copies of the HER2 gene that can lead to HER2 overexpression. In some cases, recommendations for special targeted biological therapy are advised as part of your treatment.

Understanding the Stage

Don't confuse stage with grade. This is a very common problem. They are quite different. *Grade*, as we just discussed, relates to cell growth. *Stage* combines several pieces of information (diameter of the tumor, nodal involvement, and other organ involvement) and is in some degree tied to survival estimates. Remember, however, that you are not a statistic. You are a person. People need to fall on both sides of the statistics to produce these numbers. You are embarking on doing whatever you need to do to be on the survival side.

Stage 0 is noninvasive breast cancer, or DCIS. Cancer cells are limited to the lining of the ducts and have gone no further.

Stage 1 cancer has spread from the ducts or lobules into the nearby fatty tissue of the breast. The tumor diameter is less than 2 cm (less than an inch); there is no cancer in the lymph nodes.

Stage 2 cancer has spread from the ducts or lobules into the nearby fatty tissue of the breast. The tumor diameter is between 2 and 5 cm (1–2 inches); sometimes there is lymph node involvement.

Early stage breast cancers are considered stages 0, 1, and 2.

In stage 3 the tumor may be larger than 5 cm (2 inches) and the cancer may or may not have spread to nodes, or the tumor is smaller with several nodes involved. The risk of spreading to lymph nodes and to other organs is of concern. Locally advanced breast cancer is considered stage 3.

Stage 4 is known as metastatic breast cancer. The cancer has spread from the breast and lymph nodes to other parts of the body, usually the bone, liver, lung, or brain. The presence of cancer in other organs is determined by scans and/or biopsies of these sites, where signs or symptoms are noted.

Genetics

For women with a family history of breast cancer, especially if their family members were diagnosed premenopausally and they are themselves young, the doctor might discuss considering a genetics evaluation. Twelve to fifteen percent of women diagnosed have a family history of breast cancer to some degree. When we see multiple first-degree relatives in the family diagnosed, women diagnosed young, women diagnosed with breast cancer in both breasts, men in the family diagnosed with breast cancer, or ovarian cancer in the family, there is heightened interest and speculation that the cause may be genetic.

Though it may sound simple to get a blood test and find this answer, it is more complicated than it appears to be. There are two known breast cancer genes: BRCA1 and BRCA2. Women carrying one of these genes have a considerably higher risk of getting breast cancer than the average population, which only carries a 12 percent lifetime risk of getting the disease. There are probably other genes yet to be discovered, however, that may predispose someone to get breast cancer, so testing negative for a gene today doesn't necessarily mean that you don't have a gene. Additionally, deciding what to do with this information can be a challenge for the patient. Some women want to act aggressively and have prophylactic mastectomies, removing both breasts, not just the one with the known cancer. Others want to try to hold onto that other breast for as long as possible as well as conserve the breast they have the disease in now. Guilt can accompany the results, too. The patient may carry the gene and her sisters may not. The sister is thankful to not have it but feels guilty that her loved one does. The impact the news can have for the next generation needs to be considered, too. Genetic counseling needs to happen before that blood test is done so that you and your family understand the ramifications of the results.

Decisions also need to be made as to whether you want your insurance company aware of this test result. Some women opt to pay out of pocket to have it done, and then decide based on the results whether they want to submit it to their insurance company. Why? To avoid falling into the insurance category of "pre-existing condition" clauses. If the patient opts to not be aggressive in preventative measures and later develops breast cancer again, her insurance company may label it a pre-existing condition and not cover the treatment. Some employers who foot the bill for the insurance may have access somehow to the information, and this also is of concern to some patients. So what sounds simple isn't so simple. However, it can be very valuable information for planning your treatment if you meet criteria for being evaluated for a genetic cause of your breast cancer.

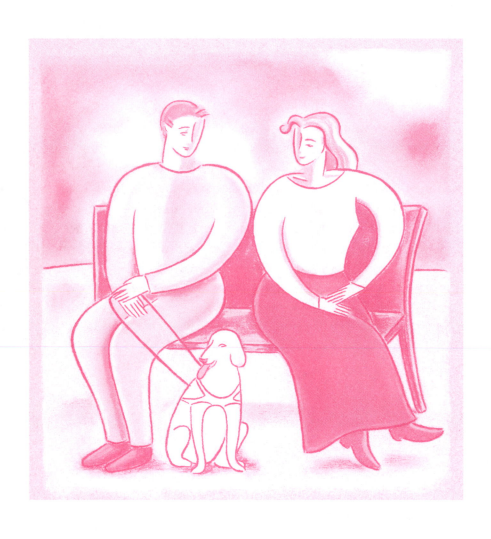

Getting Your Treatment Underway

Chapter 4

Communicating the News of the Diagnosis to Others

"Should we tell Aunt Ethel?"

Our daughter, Laura, was 12 when I was diagnosed. I was very honest with her about my diagnosis and what treatment I needed in order to be well again. She asked typical questions children ask at that age, like "Mommy, are you going to die?" and "Did you get breast cancer because you had me?" She also asked some questions I had no way of anticipating. One was, "Will the doctor move your right breast over to the middle of your chest? Because if he doesn't you are going to lean to the right when you walk." Children have a fascinating way of looking at things!

Of everyone I chose to tell, my mother was the hardest for me. I was glad I could tell her over the phone and avoid the eye contact in the process. I think that telling her I had breast cancer was like pouring acid into her ear right through the receiver of the phone. It was one of the hardest things I've ever had to communicate in my life.

Some of my friends avoided calling me after I was diagnosed because they were too upset to talk. I created a way of easing their tension by interjecting humor. I named my breast prosthesis and sent out adoption notices to my friends that I had gotten "Betty Boob."

(She was my new bosom buddy, so she deserved a name.) Soon my phone was ringing and a friend asked, "So how is Betty?" And two years later, when I was confronted with needing a second mastectomy, I called my friends and said, "I learned today that Betty Boob is getting a roommate. You need to help me choose a name for her."

—*Lillie Shockney*

When you heard the news of your diagnosis, you were in shock, right? Well, the same thing will happen to those who hear the news from you. First, decide whom you need to tell and want to tell. Those may be two different groups of people. People you need to tell are those who will be directly affected by it—family members, especially those who are now at a higher risk of getting breast cancer as a result of having a family history; your boss, who needs some information about why and when you will be taking time off from work; and your children, close friends, or others who live with you, all of whom will be very aware that something very stressful is happening that may change their routines and carry an emotional impact for them.

Telling the Children

How to tell a child his or her mother has breast cancer can be tough, no matter what the age of the child. You will need to decide if you and your partner want to tell your children together, if Mom wants to talk to the kids in private, or if Dad will deliver the news. Be honest with your children. They can read you like a book. Conspiracy breeds distrust and will make them more scared than comforted. Explain to them what will be happening in the form of treatment so that they can see you are doing something to get rid of the cancer. Many parents choose to wait to tell their children until after they've seen the doctors and know the treatment plans.

If your children are older, there may be anxiety about how this will impact them—will they get breast cancer one day, too? How will it affect their daily routines? Teens can be resentful sometimes when asked to step in and help out; it simply means that you need to know where they are coming from, mentally and emotionally. You will have to decide who will tell the kids and when, but also how much detail you want to share with them.

Telling Parents and Siblings

Telling parents is also tough. Mothers often wish that they had been the ones diagnosed. They want to try to control the situation and can't . . . and shouldn't. They will need to be given constructive ways to help because, no matter what, they will want to help you—even if you feel you don't need it.

Sisters may fear being the next one to be diagnosed in the family. They may need support and information to help them cope with their own anxiety about your diagnosis of breast cancer. Having them assist with information gathering for you can help engage them in your treatment and empower them with information that will help both of you. Keep your family members informed of how you are doing and how treatment is progressing. Rely on their support. Remember, this is a disease that affects the family. The other family members are also frightened—for you and for themselves.

Deciding Whether and How to Tell Coworkers/Friends

This is tricky. Some women and men are very open about their illnesses and family crises; others don't utter a word. This is a personal decision. You may choose to tell just a few close friends, or you may decide to go very public and take advantage of receiving lots of support. A possible pitfall with telling someone is specifically what to tell him or her and how to ensure that they understood what you said.

Telling people initially can be difficult, and it also may be difficult to keep these people informed as you move forward. You may want to assign someone to be the "information center," and provide all announcements about how you are doing, what treatment you are having, pathology results, and so on. Establishing an information contact for people to call for updates/news can help reduce the burden on you and ensure consistency in the information being provided. E-mail is a good way to make sure that everyone is receiving the same information at the same time and in the same manner, so consider gathering everyone's e-mail addresses and sending out broadcast e-mails to everyone at once. You will find it a huge time saver.

Some friends may avoid calling you. It isn't that they don't care; it's more likely that they don't know what to say, at least without crying. Let them know that even though the diagnosis is upsetting to hear, you need their support. Remember that support from others is part of the "treatment plan" for you and your partner. People will ask what they can do to help you, so be ready with a list of assignments to delegate. One day, perhaps, you will be able to reciprocate and help them in a crisis, if you haven't already.

Among the many things they can do are driving the children to school and events, running errands, making casseroles for your freezer, babysitting, adding you to prayer lists, helping with the housework, and—remember, humor builds your immune system—loaning you funny videos to watch.

Chapter 5

Breast Cancer Surgery and Sexual Intimacy

"Oops, did somebody say sex?"

My husband said women associate mastectomy surgery with an amputation of the breast, and that's wrong. He explained to me that I was undergoing "transformation surgery." The surgeon's mission was to transform me from a victim into a survivor. I was exchanging my breasts for another chance at life. That was a very fair trade, I had to agree.

A woman asked me, "Now that you've had two mastectomies without reconstruction, do you still have cleavage?" "The doctor surgically removed my cleave and left me with my age with the intent that I grow old," I replied. Another woman asked me, "Don't you get upset when you step into the shower each morning and look down and see that your breasts are gone?" I told her, "No, because when I step into the shower and look down, I only see that my cancer is gone."

My husband told me that when he holds me close our hearts touched and beat closer together. The partner needs to reassure the patient that his feelings for her and her attractiveness to him are not based on having breasts. Relationships and feelings go much deeper than that. My husband knew of my anxieties when I had to undergo a second mastectomy. He did something very clever. As a surprise, he swept me away to the Pocono Mountains, where the honeymooners go. He told me, "I've read that when you lose one of your senses, like your sense of sight or sense of smell, your other senses become more intensified. Maybe the same thing happens to your erogenous zones. It is my mission to prove this theory in the next 48 hours." And he did!

I underwent DIEP flap reconstruction a decade after my second mastectomy. It was a profound feeling to stand in the shower and rub a bar of soap across my new breasts. "The girls" and I went bra shopping when I was 6 weeks post-op. My husband told his brother "I feel like I'm sleeping with another woman and have my wife's permission." What an exciting time—to be given the opportunity to regain my silhouette and have healthy new breasts again.

—Lillie Shockney

Thinking Through Surgical Options

Society associates women's breasts with beauty, femininity, sexiness, and motherhood. We admire cleavage and promote it. Breast cancer surgery can threaten a woman's self-image. She may fear that she will feel like less of a woman and may worry even more that her partner will feel differently about her sexually. Talking through this very important issue is critical and should take place before surgery does.

The majority of women today have surgical options of lumpectomy, mastectomy, or mastectomy with breast reconstruction. In most cases, the survival rate is equal for lumpectomy with radiation and mastectomy. Factors that influence the possibility and advisability of these options are the size and location of the tumor, type of breast cancer, size of the woman's breast, possibly the age of the woman at time of diagnosis, and other prognostic factors. A woman with a large tumor compared to her breast volume usually is advised to have mastectomy surgery. Also, someone with multiple tumors in her breast occupying several different quadrants will usually be told that she is not a good candidate for breast conserving surgery.

Women undergoing mastectomy usually have options about whether they wish to have breast reconstruction. Although the decision is a personal one for a woman, it is usually made with a great deal of input from her partner. If reconstruction is an option, the surgeon will refer you to a plastic surgeon for consultation. At this point, you should be given an opportunity to review photos (torso shots) of women who have had various forms of reconstruction. Some breast centers have survivor volunteers available who can talk candidly with you about their personal experiences with the reconstruction process.

Reconstruction options include breast implants or moving fat and tissue from one part of the body to the chest to rebuild your breast. Most women are candidates for some type of reconstruction. The timing and specific type of reconstruction recommended depend on the stage and aggressiveness of the disease, the amount of fatty tissue you have, your medical history, whether radiation is needed as part of your treatment, and your thoughts about your own body image.

There is no right or wrong answer about breast reconstruction. Each woman, with her partner's input, needs to decide this for herself. You each may have assumptions about the way you feel about your breasts that surprise you. What the majority of couples quickly learn is that their priority is on surviving this disease; having breasts or not becomes a secondary issue. Because surgery is usually the first step of treatment, it is important to express your feelings and work through them.

Women commonly want to rush through treatment and not do reconstruction. They are so focused on survival that they short-change themselves. It has been said that women need permission to choose reconstruction, and from my experience that is true. Reconstruction does not delay your treatment or affect your long-term survival outcome. It also doesn't make it more difficult to diagnose a recurrence, a common concern women have. So explore your options and think about how you want to look and feel a year from now. Don't be focusing solely on rushing through to get to the finish line. A short-term investment in time to have reconstruction can be one of the most important things you do for yourself along this journey of treatment. Don't worry about insurance coverage for this. Thanks to the Women's Health and Cancer Rights Act, passed in October 1998, reconstruction is covered by your health insurance.

Women who desire immediate reconstruction but are not, for medical reasons, good candidates for the procedure need to find peace within themselves about the situation. Talking with other breast cancer survivors who have experienced the same situation can be very helpful and enlightening. Your health care team can connect you with a local support group.

The following are types of breast cancer surgery that may be discussed with you:

- *Lumpectomy*—Removal of the tumor in the breast with a margin of healthy tissue around it in all directions; also known as breast conserving surgery or partial mastectomy. Recovery time is usually just a few days.

- *Sentinel node biopsy*—The sentinel node is also known as the guard node. It is considered the first node in the armpit area (axillae) that would be affected by cancer, so if the cancer were to spread from the breast to the axillary nodes it would go to this node first. This node is identified by use of a special blue dye or a radioactive isotope injected before the surgery is begun (also known as sentinel node mapping). There can be several sentinel nodes, but most of the time there is one. This single node is removed and sent to pathology to determine if there is cancer in the node. If there is no cancer, then the rest of the nodes can be left alone because the risk of there being cancer in other nodes is extremely low. This procedure, now a standard of care, dramatically reduces the risk of lymphedema and other arm problems associated with axillary node dissections. A separate incision, very small, just below the hair line in your armpit is made to access and view this sentinel node and remove it.

- *Total simple mastectomy*—Removal of the breast, nipple, and areola. No lymph nodes from the axillae are taken. Recovery from this procedure, if no reconstruction is done at the same time, is usually 1–2 weeks. Hospitalization varies—for some it may be an outpatient procedure and for others it may require an overnight stay.

- *Axillary node dissection*—Lymph nodes serve as a filtering system for the lymphatic system (a system of vessels that collects fluids from cells for filtration and reentry into the blood). Axillary dissection is surgically explained in terms of three levels. Level I axillary dissection is also called lower axillary dissection because it is the removal of all tissue below the axillary vein and extending to the side where the axillary vein crosses the tendon of a muscle called the latissimus dorsi. Level II dissection removes diseased tissues deeper in the middle (medial) area of another muscle called the pectoralis minor. Level III dissection is the most aggressive breast cancer axillary surgery, and it involves the removal of all nodal tissue from the axilla.

If the sentinel node is determined to contain cancer cells or if ultrasound followed by a fine needle biopsy has confirmed involvement of the nodes, the surgeon will perform an axillary node dissection, which includes removal usually of level 1 and sometimes level 2 nodes. There are three levels of nodes. Most of the time level 3 is left alone. Axillary node dissection helps to plan the staging information of the disease when one node has already been confirmed to contain cancer. The risk of lymphedema increases when there is a need to dissect these nodes. Getting instructions about ways to reduce this risk is important and should be reviewed with you prior to surgery. Most women having axillary node dissections do not ever develop lymphedema, however. A separate incision is made to remove these nodes. Range of motion and arm strength usually are regained in 2–3 weeks. This procedure is generally done as an ambulatory surgery procedure.

- *Modified radical mastectomy*—This procedure is removal of the breast, nipple, and areola as well as axillary node dissection. Recovery, when surgery is done without reconstruction, is usually 3–4 weeks.

- *Skin-sparing mastectomy*—This is the removal of the breast, nipple, and areola, keeping the outer skin of the breast intact. It is a special method of performing a mastectomy that allows for good cosmetic outcome when combined with reconstruction done at the same time.

- *Breast implant reconstruction*—Usually at time of mastectomy a tissue expander is placed underneath the chest muscle and over a period of several weeks is expanded. Once it has reached the expansion size desired, the tissue expander is removed and replaced with a permanent implant. Implants can be silicone, saline, or a combination of both. Hospitalization usually is overnight, and recovery takes 2–3 weeks. There is some discomfort with the expansion process because it is stretching the chest muscle.

- *TRAM flap reconstruction*—Taking the tummy tissue and fat along with the muscle that provides the blood supply and tunneling the tissue up to the chest to rebuild the breast, forming a mound. Hospitalization is commonly 4–6 nights and recovery is 6–8 weeks due to the muscle being taken. There is a risk of hernia later with this method due to muscle loss. If done bilaterally, the risk of hernia can be high. Women are discouraged from heavy lifting short and long term. Does result in a tummy tuck.

- *Latissimus dorsi flap reconstruction*—Taking the tissue, fat, and muscle from under the shoulder blade and bringing it around to the front to rebuild the breast. Hospitalization is usually 3–5 days and the recovery period is 5–6 weeks. Some women report difficulty doing rigorous exercise that involves this muscle, such as swimming and golfing.

- *DIEP flap reconstruction (deep inferior epigastric perforator flap)*—This involves taking the tummy tissue and fat but no muscle. The doctor must identify one of the tiny perforator vessels in the muscle, tease it out of the muscle leaving the muscle wall intact, cut the tissue free from the body, and transplant this tissue and fat up to the chest to rebuild the breast. It requires a microvascular procedure to reconnect the blood vessel in the chest area. This is a highly technical procedure that requires a microscope to reconnect the vascular supply. Hospitalization is 3–4 days; recovery is 4–5 weeks. No lifting restrictions are usually imposed because muscle has not been sacrificed. Also results in a tummy tuck.

- *S-GAP reconstruction*—Taking the gluteal fat from the buttocks to rebuild the breast. Requires microvascular surgery to reconnect the blood vessels. Hospitalization is 3–4 days. Recovery usually takes 3–4 weeks. This surgery is not commonly done, usually only if the patient wants a tissue transfer and doesn't have adequate tummy fat.

- *Nipple reconstruction*—This procedure is generally done several months after the reconstruction of the breast so that the tissue/implant has "settled in." This helps ensure accurate placement of the nipple. It is done as an outpatient procedure and the breast mound is used to create the nipple projection. This reconstructed nipple will not have sensation or change in its appearance from stimulation or temperature change. No real recovery time is needed. Local anesthetic is given for the procedure. No compression of the newly built nipple is to be done for 2 weeks.

- *Areola tattooing*—Organic tattoo dye is used to create an areola. Commonly this is done by a nurse practitioner or physician's assistant in the doctor's office. The diameter and pallet shade is based on matching the other remaining breast. If the patient is undergoing bilateral areola tattooing then she can choose her diameter and color. This procedure takes approximately 30 minutes. There can be some fading of the color, requiring it to be touched up later. No recovery time is needed. Keeping it dry and clean during healing is important. Women are discouraged from going to a tattoo parlor to have this done. The tattoo dye substance is different. Dye in parlors contains lead that could appear as an abnormality on an MRI if one is needed.

Once the decision is finally made about what treatment plan is best for you, you will feel better. You will now be taking action against the disease. No matter what surgical option is selected, on the day of surgery, focus on this being "transformation day"—you are being transformed from a breast cancer victim into a breast cancer survivor and taking your first leap upward on the survival curve.

Mastectomy surgeries as well as axillary node dissections and reconstruction procedures usually involve the placement of small drains. These are left in for several days. You will be shown by one of the nurses in the breast center how to care for your drains and incisions during the recovery process. Pertinent exercises will also be shown to you to get range of motion and body strength back on track.

If you are embarking on a mastectomy without reconstruction, you will be eligible to be fitted for a breast prosthesis 6–8 weeks post-op. During the interim the doctor will give you a temporary breast form to wear in a surgical bra. When going to be fitted, seek out a mastectomy supply shop that has a certified fitter. A proper-fitting bra and prosthesis are important for balance and comfort.

Deciding who will help you at home after surgery sounds simple but sometimes isn't. You may need some assistance at home managing drains for a few days, attending to wound care and such, and recovering from surgery in general. The length of time you need help will depend on the type of surgery you have. Ask the surgeon what to expect and request to meet with the nurse to review preoperative teaching instructions prior to your surgery date so you are well prepared as to what to expect.

If other people will be coming to stay, talk about roles and responsibilities beforehand. Write out what each person is responsible for doing—buying the groceries, changing bandages, making dinner, taking the kids to soccer practice, and so on. Planning ahead prevents problems later. Function as a team—remember, this is a team effort!

You and your family member or friend who will be helping to take care of you need to talk about your expectations of each other. One issue that many couples encounter, for example, is when to see the incision. The woman, as the patient, needs to be in charge—you need to call the shots regarding the timing of when you are comfortable with showing your incision to your partner. How he looks at you and what he says the first time will stay with you the rest of your life. Some women are comfortable right away; others delay for some time. Don't delay too long, though. It is advisable to talk about this in advance and agree on a plan.

If your surgery involves drains and wound management at home, decide in advance who will be responsible for helping with emptying the drains and providing wound care at home. Have you seen photos to know what to expect the incision to look like? For most women undergoing lumpectomy, there will be little difference in the overall appearance of the breast. Women undergoing mastectomy without reconstruction will look like a young girl again, with a smooth flat chest on one side. For women undergoing reconstruction, it will be important to look at it as a work in progress, because reconstruction takes several episodes of surgical treatment before it is perfected.

Resuming Physical Intimacy After Surgery— Is Dr. Ruth Around?

Very soon after you are home from the hospital, no matter what type of surgery you have performed, your doctor will instruct you to do a specific set of exercises to begin regaining arm strength and range of motion. This is especially important because the majority of women undergoing breast cancer surgery have one or more lymph nodes under the arm removed as part of the procedure. If you have had flap reconstruction, there will be additional exercises to regain abdominal strength and motion.

A nice way to begin resuming closeness is to have your partner help you with your arm exercises. A slow dance and some romantic music are perfect for this purpose. Consider it part of your exercise routine. During your first song you may have your hands resting on his shoulders, and by the third song, they may be up and crossed around his neck. Pick out your favorite slow dances now!

The timing of when the doctor gives you the green light to resume sexual activities will vary depending on the type of surgery you have undergone. The time frame is usually quite short for women under-going lumpectomy or mastectomy without reconstruction. With reconstructive surgery, however, you should ask your surgeon about what physical activities, including sex, can be resumed and when.

Your body and most specifically one of your erogenous zones has experienced a change. Get to know your body again and let your partner explore this with you. Men can be lost for words and not know what to say. They wonder if it's okay to touch your incision. They don't want to cause discomfort. Let your partner know what you want. Being silent usually is not helpful.

Chapter 6

Adjuvant Treatment After Surgery

"Chemotherapy, radiation therapy, hormonal therapy—golly— I may need psychotherapy before I'm through!"

I saw a cartoon of a patient sitting in his doctor's office. The patient had huge webbed ears and antennae coming from the top of his head. The doctor said, "As you will recall, I did mention possible side effects from this treatment." Well, undergoing the additional treatment needed to help restore a state of wellness—whether it be chemotherapy, radiation therapy, targeted biological therapy, or hormonal therapy—comes with side effects. But staying focused on what the treatment is for helps you endure them. Knowing that there is a beginning and an end to treatment helped me, too. I can deal with anything when I know it lasts for only a finite period of time.

—Lillie Shockney

The need for additional treatment in the form of chemotherapy, radiation therapy, targeted biological therapy, or hormonal therapy will depend on the stage of the disease, the type of surgery performed, the grade of the cancer cells, the age of the patient, and other prognostic factors determined by the pathologist after examining the breast cancer tissue itself.

It is routine and expected that women undergoing lumpectomy surgery will need radiation therapy of the conserved breast to help ensure that the cancer does not return. Approximately 70 percent of women will be advised to receive some form of chemotherapy as well. Hormonal therapy is recommended 50 percent of the time to patients to reduce the risk of recurrence of breast cancer for women whose cancer cells were hormone receptor positive.

When we actually look at the entire treatment experience from beginning to end for women needing surgery, chemo, and radiation, it lasts about 9 months on average—the same length of time it takes to conceive a child and give birth to it. That is the best way to look at your breast cancer treatment, too—you are being reborn a healthier woman.

If Chemotherapy Is Part of the Game Plan

As mentioned earlier, sometimes chemotherapy is actually recommended as the first phase of treatment against breast cancer. In such cases, it is referred to as neoadjuvant chemotherapy and is given prior to the patient undergoing surgery. The mission of the chemo in such cases is to carry the medicine to all parts of the body where the disease may be located, including beyond just the breast itself. Women with large breast tumors, or women with fairly small breasts who are hoping for lumpectomy surgery, may be advised to do chemotherapy first.

For women with early stage breast cancer, the risks and benefits need to be carefully weighed to determine if chemotherapy is wise or even necessary to do. There are many things which can help a patient and physician weigh these choices such as the size of the tumor, the stage of the breast cancer, and whether the cancer is found in the lymph nodes (See pages 28-32 regarding interpreting your pathology results). In addition, there are new tools which can add information to help this decision.

Just in the past few years, a new genomic test has been developed that can take the guesswork out of this equation for many and simplify the medical decision making by determining if the specific breast cancer cells that a patient has are the type to likely want to recur or not. This can provide a sense of emotional relief to patients—to be able to have such a test done to answer this worrisome question. Though nothing is a guarantee in life, this type of test can be an aid to the oncologist and the patient in making the decision about the benefits and risks of chemotherapy.

The test is called Onco*type* DX and is designed for women whose tumors are early stage, hormone receptor positive, HER2neu negative. This special genomic test is done on the cancer cells from the tumor tissue removed during biopsy, mastectomy or lumpectomy. Even a patient who has a relatively small tumor with a positive sentinel lymph node may meet the criteria for having this test. (In the past having a positive sentinel lymph node was almost an automatic decision maker about the need to add chemotherapy to the treatment game plan.) The results of the test are reported as a Recurrence Score between 0 and 100, which provides information about the chances that a woman's cancer will return, as well as their likelihood of benefiting from the addition of chemotherapy to hormonal therapy.

In late 2007, the American Society for Clinical Oncology (ASCO) and the National Comprehensive Cancer Network (NCCN), which are organizations that develop consensus recommendations for specific areas of cancer care, recommended the use of Onco*type* DX specifically for certain subgroups of patients with early stage, node-negative, estrogen receptor-positive breast cancer.

So ask your doctor if this is a test that may be of benefit to you in helping make your decision about adjuvant chemotherapy.

Chemotherapy, also known as a form of systemic treatment, can cause a second wave of distress due to probable hair loss, gastro-intestinal symptoms, and fatigue. Chemotherapy usually is administered intravenously and given to patients in an outpatient setting. Some protocols call for a cycle of treatment every 3 weeks; others may be more frequent. Most women undergoing chemotherapy will have treatments for 3–6 months.

Most chemotherapy regimens for breast cancer cause hair loss during treatment. Preparing in advance for this is wise. For some women this experience is more traumatic than losing part or all of their breast. Women recognize that their hair is visible to all and is also something they may take particular pride in. What to do about hair that won't be there—ideas to consider:

- Have a hair stylist cut your hair short about 10 days after the first chemo treatment (which is usually right before it will begin coming out on its own).

- Some spouses choose to shave their own heads as a symbol of support (though some men are bald already).

- Have a "coming out" party for your hair—everyone brings a hat or other head covering (scarf, turban, etc.). This is a great project for children to do for you and helps engage family members in the preparation.

- If you plan to wear a wig, go to be fitted prior to starting chemotherapy and take someone along you trust who will give you honest feedback regarding how you look. Matching your hair color and style will be easier if you go before chemo starts. (Of course, if you've always wanted to be a blonde, this might be your opportunity to test out a new look!)

- Some women opt to do a buzz cut in advance of hair loss, truly taking control of the situation. Wearing a turban or scarf is also an option, as is just plain being bald. It is your choice. During the winter months, however, do wear knitted caps while outdoors or exposed to the elements. We lose 80 percent of our body heat from the top of our head. You need to stay bundled up and warm.

- Most insurance companies will cover wigs up to $350 if submitted on a prescription as a skull prosthesis by your medical oncologist, so inquire about this.

Talk with the medical oncologist about what steps can be taken to reduce possible side effects from chemotherapy. Not everyone experiences nausea from chemotherapy. New drugs are now available to prevent or dramatically reduce nausea. Also, not all chemotherapy drugs cause hair loss. And exercise has been proven in clinical trials to help reduce the fatigue that is brought about by chemotherapy.

Focus on what chemotherapy is designed to do—destroy any cancer cells that may have spread elsewhere in the body. Use visual imagery to picture how these drugs work, and focus on those images while actually receiving the drugs.

You usually feel well the day of treatment. If side effects are to occur, they most commonly happen the night of chemotherapy or the next day. Celebrate the completion of each chemotherapy cycle. You are climbing that much higher up the survival curve with every treatment. Take pride in your victory. Enjoy the moment. It's important to realize that some patients may react differently to chemotherapy than other patients. Talking with other breast cancer survivors who have had the same chemotherapy drugs will not really answer the question for you in advance exactly how you are going to feel and what side effects you may or may not experience.

Women want to know which chemotherapy drugs work best. Your medical oncologist will review your drug options with you based on the prognostic factors learned from your pathology as well as from any scans he or she may have done in advance of your treatment. There are a variety of drug choices today, usually given in some combination with one another.

Anticipate that your doctor will discuss what clinical trials you may be a candidate for. Clinical trials are research studies in which people agree to try new therapies (under careful supervision) in order to help doctors identify the best treatments with the fewest side effects. These studies help improve the overall standard of care. Clinical trials may provide you an edge over standard treatment and in the future may actually become the new method of treatment.

If Radiation Is Part of the Game Plan

For women undergoing lumpectomy surgery, or if pathology has confirmed there are cancer cells present in several lymph nodes, or the breast tumor was large, radiation will probably be recommended. There have been vast improvements in radiation therapy, also known as local therapy, over the last two decades. Special technology is used so that only tissues that need to be radiated are radiated. Although there is some risk of radiation side effects for heart and lung tissue, this risk is markedly less today than it was in years past.

For women undergoing lumpectomy, radiation may make the breast a little pink and puffy. Some women comment that their breast is tender in a way that is similar to premenstrual tenderness. Treatments are daily (Monday through Friday), usually for 5–7 weeks. Although it means going every day to the health care facility, you are in and out quickly, usually in less than half an hour.

Radiation doesn't hurt: It feels similar to getting an X-ray, which means you don't feel a thing. However, radiation is cumulative; that's why you start getting fatigued toward the end of the treatment series.

The breast area, chest wall, and axillary area are exposed during this treatment, but you are behind closed doors with just your treatment team looking in on you. Before radiation begins, you will have some special measurements done, called simulation, to ensure that the radiation beams are always lined up the exact same way to radiate the same area consistently. A few tiny tattoo marks (little blue dots) will be made on your chest as part of the preparation process. These dots are usually permanent. Some women have become creative once treatment is completed and use one of the dots as the center of an artistic tattoo, such as a butterfly, pink ribbon, or some other symbol of significance. Just as your incision is a battle scar of courage, so are these tiny tattoo dots.

Fatigue is the most common symptom that patients report, usually occurring toward the end of the treatment experience. Feeling the need to take a nap each day during the last 2 weeks and for several weeks after completing the treatment is not unusual.

There are some ongoing clinical trials for doing radiation a bit differently than the traditional external beam radiation most commonly used. These include accelerated radiation where the patient receives radiation twice a day for 2 to 3 weeks. Brachytherapy is also being used in research trials; it involves the insertion of a balloon during lumpectomy surgery. Radiation rods or seeds are later inserted or radiation rods are inserted surgically to provide radiation treatment in less than 10 days. There are pros and cons to each method for you to discuss with your radiation oncologist.

If Hormonal Therapy Is Part of the Game Plan

Your doctor will determine if it will be advisable for you to take hormonal therapy. Hormonal therapy is totally different than hormone replacement therapy. Hormonal therapy, in the form of a SERM (selective estrogen receptor modulator) or AIs (aromatase inhibitors), helps to block the ability of estrogen to reach a breast cancer cell. If your hormone receptor test was positive, that tells the doctors that estrogen and/or progesterone may promote the growth of breast cancer cells in your body. By taking a drug that works on breast cancer cells like an estrogen blocker, the risk of cancer recurring or possibly continuing to grow is reduced. The treatment is in the form of a pill that is taken daily for 5 to 10 years. Side effects are similar to menopause, but there are other possible side effects that your doctor will discuss with you depending on the drugs recommended for you.

Hormonal therapy is a long-term commitment on your part. Due to the rapid developments researchers are making in hormonal therapy, you may be advised to take some form of hormonal therapy for as long as 10 years. When a woman is dealing with side effects from taking a medication, there can be issues with adherence to the daily schedule of taking the drug. Speak up and make your oncologist aware of any side effects you are experiencing that are influencing your decision to consider discontinuing the medication or self-adjusting the dosage. The dosage and frequency for taking the medication has been determined based on extensive research. Altering this schedule may influence the benefit you are (or aren't) receiving from this therapy. Its purpose is to reduce the risk of recurrence of this disease for you. There are medications or other over-the-counter treatments (such as vaginal lubricants) that can be used to counteract some side effects. If you are taking an aromatase inhibitor (AI), discuss with your doctor the need to get a bone density study as a baseline when you start taking the AI and periodically repeat this test to ensure your bone health is being maintained.

In the Event the Cancer Has Spread

In some cases, the doctors may discover that the cancer has spread beyond the breast to another part of the body such as the lung, bone, or liver (called metastatic breast cancer), and additional treatment may be advised. The goal then will be to get the disease under control so that your body can live in relative harmony with it. New drug therapies, specifically developed to shrink tumors and achieve a state of dormancy, are now available, and they provide women a better quality of life under such circumstances than ever before.

Chapter 7

Changes in Daily Routines

"Did anyone remember to pick up dinner?"

Writing out a plan of who would do what, when, where, and how gave me comfort. I like to be organized. Though it was hard to accept help, in retrospect, it was one of the best things I did for myself and for my family. Creating this plan also helped me regain control of my situation. I could remain in charge and feel confident that what needed to be done, at work and at home, was being handled well on my behalf.

—*Lillie Shockney*

Women are used to being the caregiver, not the one needing care. We are the schedule juggler, nurse, financial manager, babysitter, counselor, chauffeur, and magician in the family most of the time. For this reason, women sometimes aren't good at asking for and accepting help from others. Breast cancer treatment is going to alter roles, play havoc with schedules, and create additional stress for the patient, other family members, and friends helping during this time. It is inevitable.

Patients with children especially may experience a variety of role changes. Daddy may be putting young children to bed because mommy doesn't feel well tonight. Older children may be asked to help with meal preparation or laundry. It's important for you and your family to talk about your schedules and how treatment needs will impact them, and to design a new schedule to best meet your needs and those of your loved ones—with as little change as possible.

This is also the time to ask for and accept help from other family members, neighbors, and friends. After all, one day they may need your help in a very similar way.

Planning Schedules for Children

Try to maintain your children's routines as much as possible. Change creates stress no matter what the age. Even an infant who is fed an hour later than usual expresses his opinions about his altered schedule. Let your children know in advance if there will be a change in their routine. Keep children informed about what is happening related to treatment. Encourage them to help and play an active role in the treatment, too. Have younger children (ages 6 to 12) go with you to the hospital when you get one of your chemo treatments to better understand what is happening. Ask them how they picture the chemotherapy traveling through your veins destroying any bad cells that might be lingering somewhere. Have them draw special pictures to cheer you up and open your get-well cards when the mail arrives. Explain why you don't feel well and the importance of playing quietly on certain treatment days. Let young children know that they can't catch breast cancer and also aren't in any way the cause of it either.

Planning Schedules for Yourselves

Make a chart of when your treatments will be. See about having chemotherapy appointments toward the end of the week so you can have the weekend to rest up (when there will be additional help around the house). Decide if you want someone to go with you for your chemotherapy treatments. You will be at the health care facility for several hours, so plan accordingly. The day needs to be as laid back as possible for you. Depending on who is available to help and what your schedules end up being, you may decide the chemo days are "pizza night" for the kids or to pull the casserole your neighbor made out of the freezer.

For radiation, consider scheduling it at the very beginning of the day or end of the day rather than in the middle. Since this treatment is daily, you will want it to cause as little disruption to your daily routine as possible. During the last 2 weeks, you will feel more tired than usual. Factor that into your schedule and don't plan a family outing during that time or engage in any strenuous activities; get extra sleep.

Finding Private Time

In our daily lives, it is hard even in the best of circumstances for women to find private time alone, except perhaps in bed in the late evening when we often are too tired to focus on our needs.

But now, more than ever before, you need to have some high-quality time for yourself and with individuals you love. You need to talk about what is happening, discuss your fears candidly with someone you trust, and talk about what you are feeling and how you are coping with this journey you are experiencing. Most individuals personally touched by breast cancer will find themselves reassessing their values and priorities in life. Get in touch with who you really are and what you want to accomplish in your lifetime. Mortality becomes so real now, when perhaps it wasn't before. The closeness that you share with others now can be priceless moments. It is sad that it sometimes takes a diagnosis of breast cancer to serve as the catalyst for creating such moments, but that doesn't detract in any way from their beauty.

So take advantage of whatever moments you can steal and savor. In fact, plan for them to happen. Take a 20-minute walk together after dinner. The dishes can wait. Sometimes talking isn't even necessary—just being "in the moment" is enough. Consider keeping a journal of your thoughts. Even writing just two sentences a day can be very therapeutic for you.

Chapter 8

Targeted Therapy

"You got breast cancer just in time for some major breakthroughs in treatment."

In recent years, clinical trials have been completed that evaluated the effect of biological therapy. Rather than using chemotherapy, or in some cases using it in combination with chemotherapy agents, drugs that are referred to as targeted therapy are being used. A prognostic factor that pathology determines at time of surgery (see page 19 in Chapter 2) is called the HER2neu receptor. HER2neu stands for human epidermal growth receptor 2. It is a gene that helps control how cells grow, divide and repair themselves. The HER2 gene directs the production of special proteins that are called HER2 receptors. Each healthy breast cell contains two copies of the HER2 gene. This gene is designed to help cells grow normally. If a cell however has too many copies of the HER2 gene, it can result in too much HER2 protein being produced. This may result in the normal breast cell turning into a cancer cell and in determining how aggressive those cancer cells are.

To explain this further, in normal cells, the HER2 protein combines with other proteins to transmit growth signals from outside the cell to the center of the cell. If the growth signal is strong, the cell gets the message to subdivide. In cancer cells with too much HER2, a growth signal is continuously being sent from the HER2 protein, resulting in tumors growing more rapidly.

The pathologist has two approved methods for testing the HER2neu receptors. IHC (known as the DAKO HerceptTest) and FISH (Vysis PathVysion). IHC, ImmunoHistoChemistry, measures the HER2 protein (called HER2 receptor) on the surface of the cell. If it is increased, it is said to be overexpressed. The results of this test are reported as 0, 1+, 2+, or 3+. If the result is 3+, then the breast cancer is considered HER2neu positive. If the result is a score of 2+, this is considered borderline and should be retested by the FISH method. The FISH test (Fluorescence In Situ Hybridization) detects if there are too many copies of the gene. This means that the cancer cells have the capacity to make too much of the HER2n receptor protein making the cancer cells in some cases less likely to respond to certain types of treatments. Studies show that 20–25% of breast cancer patients have tumors that are HER2neu positive.

A drug called Herceptin (trastuzumab) is now in use as a biologic therapy. It is also a monoclonal antibody and in general is a more targeted form of therapy than chemotherapy. Antibodies are a part of the body's immune defense against invaders such as cancer cells. Monoclonal antibodies are mass produced in a laboratory from a single cell (or clone of cells) and are directed against a single target. This drug binds to the HER2 receptors on the surface of cells. This helps to limit the cancer cell's ability to continue to grow and subdivide. The presence of HER2 antibodies on the cancer cell itself identifies it to be an abnormal cell and directs the body's immune system to destroy the cell. Thus it works in three different ways—it may block tumor cell growth; it may target the cell for destruction by the immune system itself; or it may work with chemotherapy (paclitaxel) to destroy the HER2 positive cancer cells.

Herceptin (trastuzumab) therefore may be given alone or with chemotherapy (paclitaxel) to work differently but cooperatively to treat breast cancer. When Herceptin (trastuzumab) is used with chemotherapy that attacks and damages the DNA at the cellular level, Herceptin (trastuzumab) stops the cells from repairing themselves. Because the cells can't repair, they spontaneously die. This further slows the growth of tumor cells. Additional research is underway to see in what additional ways Herceptin (trastuzumab) can work in partnership with chemotherapy drugs and other treatments in the fight against this disease.

Women may be advised to take Herceptin (trastuzumab) for an extended period of time—a year. It is common to recommend treatments weekly. Just as is the case with any drug, women are monitored closely during administration of the drug, focusing closely on the initial IV treatments. Blood work is checked periodically and special tests are done to monitor the heart. Even though a year may seem like a long time, women are able to maintain their daily routines, including working full time. It does not cause hair loss more commonly associated with chemotherapy. Remember, it works differently—biologically. It is not side effect free however and your doctor will review with you what potential side effects you may experience if you are advised to take this type of therapy. Special cardiac studies are commonly done before beginning this type of therapy as well as during treatment. Some people who receive Herceptin therapy may develop heart problems, including congestive heart failure. The risk of these heart problems is higher in people who receive both Herceptin and chemotherapy, compared to people who receive chemotherapy alone. Your doctor may consider stopping Herceptin temporarily or permanently if you develop significantly reduced heart function. Severe allergic reactions, infusion reactions, and lung problems, including pneumonitis (inflammation of the lungs), have been seen. Rarely, these side effects have been fatal. Your doctor may consider stopping Herceptin if you begin to have severe allergic reaction, swelling, or lung problems, including trouble breathing and inflammation of the lungs.

To learn more about targeted therapy and how this type of treatment works, visit www.herceptin.com. There is a list of questions you can print off to take to your doctor's appointment that will help you to better understand your pathology results and how targeted therapy may play a role in your specific treatment needs.

There is another targeted therapy called Tykerb (lapatinib) which in some situations is recommended for patients. It is usually given for women who are dealing with advanced breast cancer. For women not responding to Herceptin, it can be used as a second option to try for women with HER2neu positive disease that has spread to other organs. It is a special drug in that it can cross the blood brain barrier to reach the brain where cancer cells may have spread for women battling metastatic disease. It's taken in pill form too.

Also visit www.breastcancer.org for information on targeted biological therapies.

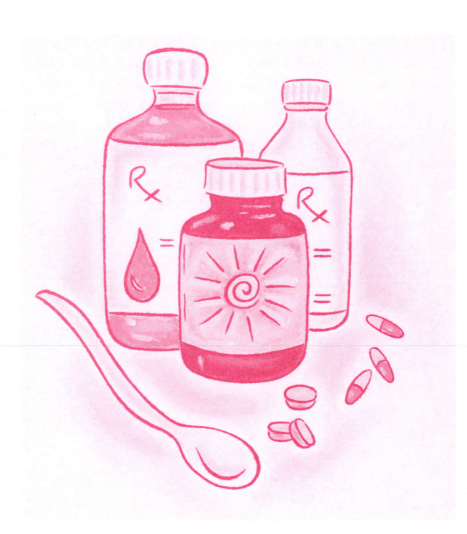

Breast Cancer as a Chronic Illness

Chapter 9

Metastatic Disease

"The goal is living in harmony with this breast cancer being part of you."

For women diagnosed with stage IV breast cancer, their cancer has spread via the lymph nodes or bloodstream to other organs such as the bone, liver, lung, or brain. This is confirmed with scans and possibly tissue biopsies. Although survival is harder to accomplish, women have managed to live in harmony with this disease for extended periods of time. That is the mission: to treat the disease like a chronic illness. If you know someone who is a brittle diabetic then you know that she takes insulin daily, usually several times a day. If she didn't, within a few days she would develop complications from her diabetes and could pass away. The mission is control of the disease. The case is the same for metastatic breast cancer.

It is not unusual for the first arm of defense against the disease to be hormonal therapy for women who are hormone receptor positive. This can be frustrating to a patient who feels she wants to be more aggressive with the disease than "just taking a pill." Talk with the doctors about the rationale for you and the approach you and your health care team want to take in getting the disease under control. Sometimes we underestimate the power of a pill. (Yet we don't question the benefits of taking a single aspirin to save our life if experiencing symptoms of a heart attack.) The bottom line: More treatment doesn't necessarily mean better treatment in fighting metastatic disease. The symptoms a patient manifests weigh heavily in the approach taken from a treatment perspective.

Usually how a patient feels is considered a good measurement as to how she actually is doing. Don't get frustrated that you aren't being scanned frequently. Cancer doesn't grow quite that fast. And remember, the mission is to get it under control so that your body lives in harmony with it.

There are specific clinical trials for women dealing with metastatic breast cancer. There are also clinical trials for women whose disease is stable, with the goal that vaccines will be developed as part of the treatment and prevention of this disease in the future.

Chapter 10

Financial Issues

"Does my insurance cover that?"

My dad's initial reaction when he learned I had breast cancer was to offer me money. He said "You will have a lot of extra expenses now. I don't want you to be worrying about finances. Worrying about cancer is enough."

This was his way to try to help. He was pleased to learn, though, that he had taught me well. We were financially stable; I had short- and long-term disability insurance and a lot of sick-leave days available. Keeping track of hospital bills, though, required organization on my part. I also called my health insurance company to find out whether some of the things that I knew I would need—like breast prostheses, mastectomy bras, and outpatient treatments—would be covered.

—*Lillie Shockney*

Dealing with breast cancer is hard enough by itself. Unfortunately, other issues such as finances, health insurance, and time lost from work can add to your stress and frustration. Words like "co-payments," "deductibles," "noncovered benefits," and "zero-balance sick leave" all conspire to complicate the cancer treatment and trying to get well. There are resources to help with these issues though, so don't go it alone.

The type of surgery you have will determine the amount of time you will need to recuperate. Women who have lumpectomy surgery are often back to their routines in 1–2 weeks. The same is true for women having a mastectomy without reconstruction. Some women resume going to work even sooner.

Women undergoing reconstruction will experience a longer recovery period due to the nature of the plastic surgery performed. It can take 6–8 weeks to recover from TRAM flap reconstruction. These women will need more assistance at home with lifting and moving than someone without breast reconstruction. Recovery from a DIEP flap typically takes 4–6 weeks, a shorter time frame due to not having to surgically involve the muscle or do any tunneling of tissue. Recovery from tissue expander insertion usually takes 1–3 weeks. Reconstruction is covered by health insurance today, thanks to a federal law passed in 1998 requiring it. Prior to that, breast reconstruction for women having a mastectomy due to breast cancer was actually considered cosmetic surgery. If additional surgery is needed to create the symmetry desired, it, too, is covered.

If you work outside the home and anticipate being out for an extended period of time, check with your employer about short-term and long-term disability to see what you qualify for. This coverage may help to supplement your pay considerably. Also, if married, have your spouse inquire about human resources policies at his place of employment. One of the provisions of the Family and Medical Leave Act enables spouses or other family members to work flexible schedules to accommodate the needs of family members who are ill.

Today, many women work during the majority of their chemotherapy and radiation treatment periods. Talk with your boss about working a flexible schedule to accommodate the need to leave early for radiation each afternoon or being off, say, every third Friday for chemo treatments.

Check with your insurance company about what your benefits do and do not cover. There usually is coverage for mastectomy bras, breast prostheses, and wigs, although you may need to get a prescription from the doctor for the insurance company to pick up the expense or share the cost with you. Some cancer organizations, like the American Cancer Society, provide breast prostheses and wigs free to women who qualify, including women with insurance.

Find out if you are covered for medications such as anti-nausea drugs that may be needed during chemotherapy treatment. Some insurance companies don't cover this expense, and some of these drugs are very pricey. Talk with your doctor so he or she is aware of your insurance coverage. Your doctor may be prescribing a brand-name drug when your insurance company will pay only for the generic equivalent. Some pharmaceutical companies offer assistance with prescription medicines, too. Ask the nurse working with your medical oncologists about this.

Friends and family may say to you, "Let me know how to help." Don't turn these offers away. If someone wants to make a casserole for dinner for your family, let them, and say "Thank you." This will reduce your grocery bill as well as give you more time to recuperate. If Mom wants to be your chauffeur back and forth each day for radiation, let her. It's her gasoline. If someone offers to take your car pool runs for the next few months, let them. You can reciprocate later on down the road.

Planning treatment, such as chemotherapy, around your schedule may be something to consider as well to help ease financial burdens. For example, having chemotherapy on a Friday afternoon would result in you potentially missing only half a day from work. Take advantage of Saturday and Sunday being time off when you can rest and have family support at home with the hope that you will feel well enough to return to work as usual on Monday morning. Talking with your employer about flexible schedules that may enable you to work early in the morning that day may even prevent you from losing any work hours at all.

Do keep track of your out-of-pocket expenses, though. Make a chart so that you know what is paid, what is still owed, what is covered by insurance, and what is not. Some expenses may be tax-deductible. Discuss who will be responsible for keeping track of this information. You need to know what your breast cancer treatment expenses are so that you can plan ahead. Keep a record of the time that you miss from work—especially that which is not covered by sick leave or vacation time. By keeping track of all of this information, you will be better able to manage your household budget. Some employers offer their employees the opportunity to pool their sick days or donate them to other employees at their discretion so that if someone is in need of extended leave with pay and lacks adequate sick leave on his or her own, there is a way for coworkers to help out.

If you lack health insurance, all is not lost. There are resources available for women who need help and meet certain criteria for financial assistance and coverage of their breast cancer treatment expenses. Some states even have special grants for residents for precisely this purpose. Check with the social worker at the facility where you are being treated for assistance and referrals.

There are even organizations that provide support for transportation to and from treatment visits, provide food for you and your family, and offer babysitting services for breast cancer patients. They are not located in every state, however, so it will be necessary to speak with a social worker or nurse in the breast center to find out what is available in your area.

Financial support services are not well advertised. It will require you to take the initiative to ask about them rather than waiting for someone to tell you about them. Be assertive and do this for yourself. That's why these programs exist.

Money is the primary reason family members argue. Avoid this up front by discussing the issue and planning a budget. Also ask to meet with a social worker if you have special needs that need to be addressed.

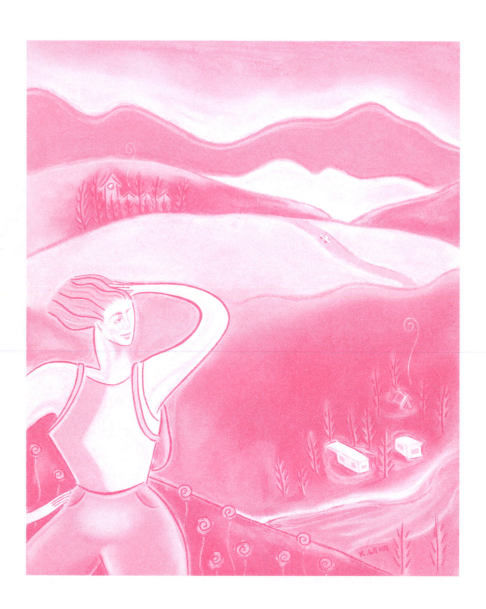

Moving Forward as a Survivor

Chapter 11

Living a Healthier Lifestyle Going Forward

"I want to feel confident I'm doing all I can to not revisit this diagnosis in my future."

Nutrition

If you eat healthier, will you prevent breast cancer? Diet does have a connection to some degree. We know that high-fat diets that encourage packing on the pounds can increase risk due to the additional weight gain (which translates into more estrogen being stored in that body fat). Eating a diet rich in green and orange vegetables is smart for your breast health as well as for your heart. This doesn't mean that you have to give up chocolate nut sundaes for the rest of your life. Eat smart. Save high-fat and high-calorie foods for special times and rewards, not daily.

If you are overweight, consider joining a group to help you reduce weight gradually. Avoid diet pills. Changing eating habits and making it part of your lifestyle is what will take the weight off and keep it off. It needs to be an overall program, not a fad diet. Women usually lose more weight when they partner with someone else working on the same goal. There is no benefit in doing this alone.

Heart-healthy menus are also breast-healthy choices.

Exercise

Muscles and bones, get ready! Exercise is a way to help reduce risk as well. Again, it helps keep your body fat to a reasonable level (rather than excessive). This doesn't mean you need to become a marathon runner and press 400 pounds at the gym. It does mean finding an exercise program that you can commit to and that makes you feel good. If you enjoy the exercise program, it is in an environment you feel comfortable in, you feel better after you do it, and it is convenient so you stick to it, then it's a winner. Power walking is one of those options. Walking three times a week for an hour will do it. Working out three times a week also will. Again, exercising with a friend usually makes it more enjoyable and helps you stick to it because you have a buddy rooting you on.

Stress

Does stress cause breast cancer? No one really knows. We do know, however, that emotional turmoil affects our immune system, and our immune system needs to be in good shape to fight cancer cells. Don't plan to sit on a beach eating bon-bons for the rest of your life, though, all because you were diagnosed with breast cancer. You will be expected to resume your chaotic life, including family responsibilities and work duties. Reassessing how you react to stressful situations is something you can do, however. Breast cancer can teach us that we really don't have to sweat the small stuff. Making time for ourselves is important, including after treatment is done. Put things into perspective before reacting to them. Is it really a crisis that your mother-in-law came over and you haven't vacuumed the floors yet? (When she rings the doorbell, grab the vacuum and put it in the middle of the living room floor. It will look like you are about to get underway even if you aren't.) Again, don't sweat the small stuff. You've been through big stuff. Learning deep breathing techniques, taking a yoga class, or doing other forms of relaxation therapy can help you in times you least expect.

Stay Informed

Remain educated about new discoveries related to this disease— don't think that because you are finished treatment you can stop reading about breast cancer. Actually, reading about cutting-edge discoveries afterward can be equally important for you. You want to "stay abreast" of the information. It is important to stay empowered for yourself and for your family members. Rely on specific sources for reliable information and not the magazines at the grocery check-out. I have provided a list of these resources for you in Chapter 14.

Chapter 12

Celebrating Completion of Breast Cancer Treatment: Survivorship

"Is our journey completed?"

One of my greatest joys is helping and supporting other women who end up "wearing my bra." I used to say that I help others who walk in my footsteps, but let's face it, I didn't have foot surgery. Each new breast cancer patient whom I help along her journey also helps me, because emotional recovery from a diagnosis of breast cancer can take a lifetime. Helping others is a key part of the healing. Having undergone lumpectomy, mastectomies, adjuvant therapy, and delayed DIEP flap reconstruction, I am able to walk the walk and talk the talk.

—*Lillie Shockney*

Although we each anticipate our treatment being completed and look forward to the day when it is, some women feel like they are still in limbo when that day actually comes. Maybe it's because our bodies aren't yet shouting to us confidently: "I am cancer free!" Maybe it's because we developed a comfort level in having doctors and nurses looking at us, poking at us, and checking on us to make sure we were "doing okay." And now, with treatment ending, that, too, is ending. Maybe it's the reality of what we have been through that sends us into a whirlwind of emotions.

Whatever its cause, it is common for women to have such emotions and develop such fears. It sometimes is referred to as "post-treatment syndrome." While we were getting treatment, we were taking action against the disease in a tangible way—cutting it out of our bodies, treating it with chemicals, or radiating it. Although there is nothing pretty about any of the treatments themselves, they each are concrete, and known to be effective ways to get rid of cancer. Now the doctor is saying, "Go back to your life. I'll see you in a few months for a check-up."

Yikes! What if the cancer comes back? How will we know, and will we know in time? How can we pick up our lives again when we know that this experience has changed us?

Fear of recurrence, dealing with the residual side effects of treatment, and needing to find our "new normal" selves make up post-treatment syndrome. But take heart, there are things we can do to address it and come out on top.

For starters, take charge of your health by living a healthy lifestyle. A good way to start your "life after breast cancer" is to make sure you eat right, stay active, sleep adequately, reduce stress, avoid smoking environments, and capture high-quality time.

Talk with your doctor about what side effects might linger so that if you have an ache or pain a month from now, you won't panic. It is common for some side effects from chemo, such as joint pain, to remain for a while.

What are the signs and symptoms that your doctor wants you to report to him or her if they occur? Examples may be a new lump in the breast or an ache or pain that is new, remains constant, and doesn't go away after 3 weeks.

Set new goals. This is a time for reflection, a time to reassess what is really important in your life. Some people make career changes to fulfill goals they never thought possible or had planned to accomplish "some day." Decide what goals you want to accomplish. Make a list. Putting them down on paper helps to make them more tangible and will help you to work on a plan to achieve them.

The majority of breast cancer awareness events raise money for research. This is a comforting way to know you are helping to make a difference for the next generation. So participate, and walk with pride.

Get involved as a volunteer. One of the best ways to move on from your experience with breast cancer is to help those who are diagnosed after you. By helping someone else, you help yourself psychologically, because although recovery from breast cancer itself may take a finite time physically, emotional recovery can take a lifetime. Being diagnosed and treated for breast cancer is a life-altering experience. It can be life altering in a positive way if we just let it. Become a breast cancer survivor volunteer. Help your hospital benefit the next generation. Volunteer as a breast cancer survivor at the hospital where you were diagnosed and treated. By giving to others, you personally will gain a great deal.

Educate others and help promote breast cancer awareness in your local community. You can save other women's lives (and breasts) by promoting mammography, breast self-exam, and clinical breast exams. If all women over the age of 40 got an annual mammogram, the number of deaths from breast cancer each year would be reduced by one third—that's 15,000 lives a year!

One day I plan to learn ventriloquism so that my breasts can speak out to the public and, just as the crash dummies in television commercials encourage people to wear seat belts, my breasts can teach women about the value of early breast cancer detection and the importance of maintaining good breast health!

—Lillie Shockney

Chapter 13

What Does the Future Hold in the Field of Breast Cancer?

"Will there always be a need for breast cancer walks?"

Today nearly every women's magazine carries articles on breast cancer. The month of October brings literally thousands of families and friends together for breast cancer walks, races, pink ribbon awareness luncheons, and educational seminars, all targeting this disease. The goal is consistent—raise awareness, promote early detection, and raise research dollars for better treatments and an eventual cure.

There are bumper stickers that say, "Women are dying for a cure" and "Help us find a cure so our daughters don't have to." So will there ever be a cure? I confidently say "yes," not because I want it badly for my future granddaughters, but because I can see it on the horizon. When I'm feeling down because a patient I've gotten close to has succumbed to this disease, I only need to visit our Breast Cancer Research Labs at Johns Hopkins to feel hopeful for future patients.

Just since my own original diagnosis in 1992, great progress has been made:

- Sentinel node biopsy has replaced axillary node dissections, dramatically reducing risk of lymphedema.

- DIEP flap reconstruction has replaced TRAM flap, sparing abdominal muscles today.

- Targeted therapy has been developed to increase survival odds for women with aggressive, difficult to control tumors.

- Genetic testing is available for two breast cancer genes that predispose an individual to get breast cancer.

- More clinical trials have been developed and completed showing benefits of specific chemotherapy agents and what combinations may be more useful.

- Shortened radiation therapy techniques have been developed.

This is just a partial list of breakthroughs that have happened in a little more than a decade.

Other treatments now in clinical trial stages include the following:

- Newer chemotherapy combinations

- Neoadjuvant chemotherapy for even early stage breast cancers

- Laser ablation of tumors including single foci tumors of liver metastasis

- Administration of chemotherapy directly into the ducts of the breast to destroy the source of the disease

- New hormonal therapies and vaccine therapies that are being tested

We are developing a better understanding of why and how breast cancer spreads, recognizing that if we could prevent it from ever spreading, frankly no one would die of this disease.

In laboratory petri dishes breast cancer cells are being studied to further understand what stimulates them to grow and thrive. There is also exciting research looking at ways to prevent breast tissue from ever allowing cells to mutate into a breast cancer cell.

You and I have the opportunity to see, in our lifetime, this disease listed in medical books in the chapter under "cured diseases" where polio is listed today. Until then, I'll be looking for you at future breast cancer events, proudly wearing your pink hat or t-shirt proclaiming that you are, like me, a breast cancer survivor.

Chapter 14

Resources of Benefit to Breast Cancer Patients and Their Families

There is a wealth of information about breast cancer available on the Internet, in bookstores, and through various breast cancer organizations. This is a list of resources to help you focus on a few that may be of particular benefit to you and your family.

The American Cancer Society's Breast Cancer Network

American Cancer Society

800-ACS-2345

http://www.cancer.org

The American Cancer Society is a nationwide, community-based organization with chartered divisions across the country. This Web site is the home page for information about clinical research trials funded by the ACS; the Reach to Recovery program, which provides one-on-one support to newly diagnosed patients; and the American Cancer Society's free programs such as Road to Recovery, I Can Cope, and Look Good Feel Better. Also consider contacting your local ACS office for information and support.

Cancer Information Service of the National Cancer Institute

800-4-CANCER

http://www.cancer.gov

This organization provides information about all types of cancer including excellent information about breast cancer: what it is, how it is treated, and where various treatment options are provided. You can request free information by calling the toll-free number.

The Johns Hopkins Avon Foundation Breast Center

410-955-4851

410-614-2853 (Lillie Shockney's Direct Line)

Her e-mail: shockli@jhmi.edu

http://www.hopskinsbreastcenter.org

This breast center is one of the few comprehensive cancer centers in the country that offers state-of-the-art breast cancer diagnosis and treatment. A special feature online is Artemis, Hopkins's electronic breast cancer medical journal that you can subscribe to for free. It is published online monthly and provides the most up-to-date information about the latest available research results and information related to diagnosis and treatment of this disease. The Web site also has sections about diagnosis and treatment information, breast imaging, pathology and breast reconstruction, breast cancer patient bill of rights, and other valuable resource information.

If you plan to be evaluated or treated at Johns Hopkins, you will probably meet me. I interact with patients daily and match the team of breast cancer survivor volunteers with women newly diagnosed based on their age, stage of disease, and anticipated treatment plan. The survivor volunteer, who has already completed the same treatment plan the patient is about to embark on, remains connected with the patient as long as the patient desires, which usually is through and beyond the end of treatment.

Komen for the Cure

National Helpline 800-IM-AWARE

http://www.komen.org

This is a national volunteer organization seeking to eradicate breast cancer as a life-threatening disease, working through local chapters and the Race for the Cure events in more than 110 cities. The foundation is the largest private funder of breast cancer research in the United States. The Komen Alliance is a comprehensive program for the research, education, diagnosis, and treatment of breast disease. You will find information on its Web site about its mission, the accomplishments it has achieved to date, how you can participate, grants it has funded, a national calendar of events, and other information. Komen is very big on education about the disease and on ensuring treatment for the underserved.

Mothers Supporting Daughters with Breast Cancer (MSDBC)

410-778-1982

E-mail: msdbc@verizon.net

http://www.mothersdaughters.org

This is a national nonprofit organization dedicated to providing support to mothers who have daughters diagnosed with breast cancer. This organization offers a free "mother's handbook" and "daughter's companion booklet" that provide basic information about breast cancer and its treatment as well as some recommended, constructive ways for mothers to provide support physically, emotionally, financially, and spiritually. The organization also "matches" mothers with mother volunteers across the country based on the daughter's (patient's) clinical picture, age at time of diagnosis, and anticipated treatment plan. MSDBC also has a newsletter online and a bulletin board for posting questions. I'm the "daughter" and co-founder of this organization.

Herceptin.com

http://www.Herceptin.com

This Web site, supported by Genentech, provides a valuable resource online for patients and their families to understand information about biological targeted therapy as well as the basics regarding clinical trials and questions to ask about participating in clinical trials.

TheBreastCareSite.com

http://www.thebreastcaresite.com

This is a Web site sponsored by Amoena/Coloplast. It provides educational information about breast health and breast cancer, including monthly articles and an Ask the Expert section.

Y-Me National Breast Cancer Organization

800-221-2141 (24-hour national hotline)

800-221-2141 (24-hour hotline in Spanish)

E-mail: info@y-me.org

http://www.y-me.org

Y-Me is committed to providing information and support to anyone who has been touched by breast cancer. The services listed on its Web site include a national hotline for women needing emotional support, a kid's corner, referral information for approved mammography facilities near you, public education workshops where you will find a listing of upcoming events, teen programs where you can order a video specifically for teenage girls to learn about breast cancer awareness, and a resource library that provides information about treatment modalities.

Young Survival Coalition

155 6th Avenue

10th Floor

New York, NY 10013

212-206-6610

E-mail: info@youngsurvival.org

http://www.youngsurvival.org

The Young Survival Coalition (YSC) is the only international, nonprofit network of breast cancer survivors and supporters dedicated to the concerns and issues that are unique to young women and breast cancer. Through action, advocacy, and awareness, the YSC seeks to educate the medical, research, breast cancer, and legislative communities and to persuade them to address breast cancer in women 40 and under. The YSC also serves as a point of contact for young women living with breast cancer.

Breastcancer.org

http://www.breastcancer.org

Breastcancer.org is a nonprofit organization dedicated to providing the most reliable, complete, and up-to-date information about breast cancer. Its mission is to help women and their loved ones make sense of the complex medical and personal information about breast cancer, so they can make the best decisions for their lives.

Living Beyond Breast Cancer

http://www.lbbc.org

Living Beyond Breast Cancer (LBBC) is dedicated to assisting you, whether you are newly diagnosed, in treatment, recently completed treatment, are years beyond, or are living with advanced (metastatic) disease. They are also there for your family members, caregivers, friends, and healthcare providers to provide breast cancer information and support. They offer teleconferences as well as quarterly educational seminars to provide cutting edge information related to diagnosis and treatment options.

People Living With Cancer

http://www.peoplelivingwithcancer.org

People Living With Cancer, the patient information Web site of the American Society of Clinical Oncology (ASCO), is designed to help patients and families make informed healthcare decisions. The site provides information on more than 85 types of cancer, clinical trials, coping, side effects, a Find an Oncologist database, patient support organizations, and more.

Commonly Asked Questions That Perhaps You Have Wondered About

Q: Does having a breast biopsy with a needle or stereotactic method cause breast cancer to spread to other areas of the breast as the needle is withdrawn?

A: No. There was a time this was thought to be true, but it has been determined not to be so.

Q: Why can't a frozen section be done on breast tissue so that the surgeon knows in the operating room that he got it all and all the margins are clear?

A: Several decades ago frozen sections were done. It was later determined that there is a high error rate with such a technique on breast tissue because it is primarily made up of fatty cells and fat doesn't freeze and slice well. This resulted in pathology errors. That is why it was discontinued about 20 years ago. To ensure accuracy takes time and proper specimen preparation.

Q: Does taking HRT cause breast cancer?

A: Taking HRT for an extensive period of time is now considered a risk factor for getting this disease, but not actually the cause. If you are destined to get breast cancer, it may be speeding up its arrival by as much as a decade because many breast cancers are stimulated to grow with estrogen.

Q: I'm starting to get peach fuzz hair but am still taking chemotherapy. Does this mean that the chemo isn't working anymore?

A: No. Some women do report their hair attempting to regenerate itself earlier than anticipated. If you have been on one chemo agent and now are on another agent, ask if this second regimen of treatment also causes hair loss. Not all chemotherapy drugs do.

Q: Does nipple discharge mean I have breast cancer?

A: Actually, nipple discharge is more common than women may realize. Often the cause is hormonal changes. It always warrants being checked out, though, to ensure it is not something more serious.

Q: Is LCIS a form of breast cancer?

A: Though it is called lobular "carcinoma" in situ, it in fact is not breast cancer but instead is a marker for predicting risk of potentially getting the disease. This is quite different from DCIS, ductal carcinoma in situ, which is noninvasive breast cancer, Stage 0 disease.

Q: I had breast cancer 20 years ago and was treated with a mastectomy. Is it too late to consider reconstruction now?

A: It is never too late, and in the last 20 years better reconstruction techniques have been developed. See a plastic surgeon that specializes in all the methods of reconstruction to discuss the option that's best for you.

Q: It has been 10 years since my diagnosis and treatment and I still worry about the disease coming back. Will the worrying ever go away?

A: Fear of recurrence is the most common fear women have after being diagnosed and treated. The greatest risk of recurrence is in the first 2 years. The next milestone to reach is the 6-year mark. Recurrence risk dramatically declines after this. With each passing year feel more confident that you are doing well and are cancer free.

Q: Now that I'm a breast cancer survivor, should I still be followed by my regular gynecologist or see a gyn oncologist instead?

A: Though risk of other cancers like ovarian cancer is an issue for breast cancer survivors, it usually isn't necessary to see a gyn oncologist unless there is a history of ovarian cancer in the family or knowledge of a breast cancer gene predisposing you to ovarian cancer. It is important, however, to be followed by a gynecologist knowledgeable in the care of breast cancer. The issues you face in the future are different than they were before, such as menopausal management that cannot be done with HRT, the need for thorough clinical breast exams, and so on. So find out the knowledge base of your present gynecologist to determine if you need to change to someone else who may specialize in breast cancer survivors. They exist.

Where Can I Get Help with Financial or Legal Concerns?

Accompanying any serious illness are questions and concerns related to expenses incurred as a result of treatment, health insurance questions that can be overwhelming to try to understand or resolve alone, and sometimes even legal questions related to employment or financial matters. Following is a list of national resources to aid you in addressing these types of concerns.

CancerCare, Inc.

212-302-2400

800-813-HOPE

E-mail: info@cancercare.org

http://www.cancercare.org

CancerCare is a national nonprofit organization that provides free, professional assistance to people with any type of cancer and to their families. This organization offers education, one-on-one counseling, financial assistance for nonmedical expenses, and referrals to community services.

Credit Counseling Centers of America (CCC America)

800-493-2222

http://www.cccamerica.org

CCC America is a nonprofit organization that provides a wide array of consumer and creditor services for individuals and families experiencing financial distress.

Health Insurance Association of America

202-824-1600

800-879-4422

http://www.hiaa.org

HIAA is a lobbyist group for insurance companies. It can help answer questions regarding health insurance coverage.

Hill-Burton Free Care Program

800-638-0742

In Maryland call 800-492-0359

http://www.hrsa.gov/osp/dfcr

This is a national government agency that provides referrals for free medical care at participating medical facilities and most hospitals, and helps low-income individuals pay their medical bills.

National Association of Hospital Hospitality Houses, Inc.

PO Box 18087

Asheville, NC 22814-0087

828-253-1188

800-542-9730

E-mail: helpinghomes@nahhh.org

http://www.nahhh.org

NAHHH is a service organization of hospital hospitality houses (HHH). Member houses provide a variety of services—primarily no-cost or low-cost housing for families and patients requiring hospital treatment or care away from their homes. At present, there are approximately 150 HHH-type facilities in the United States and Canada.

National Coalition for Cancer Survivorship (NCCS)

301-650-8868

877-NCSS-YES

E-mail: info@cansearch.org

http://www.cansearch.org

This network of independent groups and individuals provides information and resources about cancer support, advocacy, and quality of life issues and also helps cancer patients deal with insurance or job discrimination and other related legal matters.

Patient Advocate Foundation

757-873-6668

800-532-5274

E-mail: patient@pinn.net

http://www.patientadvocate.org

This organization provides educational information about managed care/insurance issues and legal counseling on debt intervention, job discrimination issues, and insurance denials of coverage.

Social Security Administration

Office of Public Inquiries

800-772-1213

http://www.ssa.gov

The SSA is the U.S. government agency that runs the Social Security program. It can provide information about retirement and disability benefits, supplemental security income (SSI), and Medicare.